HEMOPHILIA CARE IN THE NEW MILLENNIUM

ADVANCES IN EXPERIMENTAL MEDICINE AND BIOLOGY

Recent Volumes in this Series

Volume 479
THE BIOLOGY AND PATHOLOGY OF INNATE IMMUNITY MECHANISMS
Edited by Yona Keisari and Itzhak Ofek

Volume 480
BIOLOGY OF THE MAMMARY GLAND
Edited by Jan A. Mol and Roger A. Clegg

Volume 481
ELASTIC FILAMENTS OF THE CELL
Edited by Henk L. Granzier and Gerald H. Pollack

Volume 482
CHROMOGRANINS: Functional and Clinical Aspects
Edited by Karen B. Helle and Dominique Aunis

Volume 483
TAURINE 4: Taurine and Excitable Tissues
Edited by Laura Della Corte, Ryan J. Huxtable, Giampietro Sgaragli, and Keith F. Tipton

Volume 484
PHYLOGENETIC PERSPECTIVES ON THE VERTEBRATE IMMUNE SYSTEM
Edited by Gregory Beck, Manickam Sugumaran, and Edwin L. Cooper

Volume 485
GENES AND PROTEINS UNDERLYING MICROBIAL URINARY TRACT VIRULENCE: Basic Aspects and Applications
Edited by Levente Emődy, Tibor Pál, Jörg Hacker, and Gabriele Blum-Oehler

Volume 486
PURINE AND PYRIMIDINE METABOLISM IN MAN X
Edited by Esther Zoref-Shani and Oded Sperling

Volume 487
NEUROPATHOLOGY AND GENETICS OF DEMENTIA
Edited by Markus Tolnay and Alphonse Probst

Volume 488
HEADSPACE ANALYSIS OF FOODS AND FLAVORS: Theory and Practice
Edited by Russel L. Rous

Volume 489
HEMOPHILIA CARE IN THE NEW MILLENNIUM
Edited by Dougald M. Monroe, Ulla Hedner, Maureane R. Hoffman, Claude Negrier, Geoffrey F. Savidge, and Gilbert C. White II

HEMOPHILIA CARE IN THE NEW MILLENNIUM

Edited by

Dougald M. Monroe

University of North Carolina School of Medicine
Chapel Hill, North Carolina

Ulla Hedner

Novo Nordisk A/S, Målov, Denmark and
University of Lund, Lund, Sweden

Maureane R. Hoffman

Duke University and Durham VA Medical Centers
Durham, North Carolina

Claude Negrier

Hôpital Edouard Herriot
Lyon, France

Geoffrey F. Savidge

Guys' and St. Thomas's Trust
London, United Kingdom

and

Gilbert C. White II

University of North Carolina School of Medicine
Chapel Hill, North Carolina

KLUWER ACADEMIC / PLENUM PUBLISHERS
New York, Boston, Dordrecht, London, Moscow

Library of Congress Cataloging-in-Publication Data

Hemophilia care in the new millennium / edited by Dougald M. Monroe ... [et al.].
p. cm. -- (Advances in experimental medicine and biology ; 489)
Includes bibliographical references and index.
ISBN 0-306-46521-3
1. Hemophilia--Congresses. I. Monroe, Dougald McDougald. II. Series.

RC642 .H453 2001
616.1'572--dc21

00-054579

ISBN 0-306-46521-3

233 Spring Street, New York, N.Y. 10013

http://www.wkap.nl/

10 9 8 7 6 5 4 3 2 1

A C.I.P. record for this book is available from the Library of Congress

Printed in the United States of America

PREFACE

There should be, and in the best of cases there is, a synergy between basic research and patient care. However, this synergy is hard to develop because the techniques required to be a successful researcher are so different from the skills required to be an outstanding physician. Harold R. Roberts, M.D., of the University of North Carolina at Chapel Hill, is an example of a physician-researcher who has benefited from having his feet in both the world of patient care and the world of the laboratory: he has let clinical problems direct his basic research effort and conversely has adopted research advances in his care of patients.

Dr. Roberts's long and continuing career has included many research and clinical advances. He was part of the first group to determine the amino acid sequence of the important thrombin inhibitor hirudin and part of the group that prepared the first cryoprecipitates which were the first alternative to plasma as therapy in hemophilia A. Dr. Roberts has made significant advances in understanding the protein chemistry behind hemophilia B; he was among the first researchers to identify some patients as not being completely deficient but instead as having measurable levels of protein and subsequently demonstrated that this protein was dysfunctional. This important advance led him to a classification scheme for patients into Cross Reacting Material (CRM) positive, negative, and reduced. Dr. Roberts was the first to identify the molecular defect in a hemophilia B patient (factor IX Chapel Hill). He was the first to identify defects in factor IX activation and his group was one of the first to develop recombinant factor IX molecules with significantly enhanced activity. His contributions as a physician are also numerous. He was one of the first to argue for strong viral inactivation procedures in the product supply. He was one of the first to treat patients with high purity factor concentrates, recombinant factor concentrates (both hemophilia A and B) and with high-dose recombinant factor VIIa. He also conducted important research studies on the mechanism behind the action of high dose factor VIIa.

He has encouraged the exchange of information between scientists internationally as the executive director of the International Society for Thrombosis and Hemostasis and in 1978 he established the UNC-CH Center for Thrombosis and

Hemostasis to encourage collaborations among scientists at the University of North Carolina at Chapel Hill.

Advances in both patient care and research have been rapid in the twentieth century. Planners of the "Hemophilia Care in the New Millennium" symposium, held in Chapel Hill on April 8-10, 1999, felt that on the eve of a new century it was urgent to bring together physicians and researchers to look at four important areas which are at the crossroads between patient care and research.

The symposium and this book are dedicated to Dr. Roberts in honor of his many and continuing contributions to the field.

In this book, part I explores transmissible agents, especially viral agents, as a risk to the blood supply. The chapter in this section describes the major viruses that are transmitted as a consequence of transfusion. The chapter describes the incidence of these viruses and presents information about the screening tests that are available. This summary shows that current methods of viral inactivation have so far proven quite effective and should, with due diligence, prove effective in the future. However, the question of how to prevent transmission of infectious agents hidden in cells has arisen. This chapter touches on current research into ways of inactivating such transmissible agents. These studies may ultimately be brought to the clinical setting to provide a safer blood supply.

In part II, Unexplained Aspects of Hemophilia and Hemostasis, the two chapters look at clinical problems that present puzzles to researchers. These types of problems provide some of the strongest rational for interaction between clinicians and researchers. For example, protein S deficiency is clearly associated with thrombotic complications in patients, yet assays commonly used in the research laboratories have not unambiguously identified a mechanism for the action of protein S. In this book, Dr. Nurden and colleagues form a clinical question by combining two observations: 1) platelet aggregation appears to be important in the development of atherosclerotic lesions and 2) some patients have platelet defects such that their platelets do not aggregate. The investigators then pose the question: do these defects protect patients from atherosclerosis? Also in this section, Dr. Kalafatis and Dr. Mann give an overview of the function of factor V. Since mutation of a specific residue of factor V, residue 506, leads to a common mutation called factor V Leiden, and since activated protein C cleaves factor V at this residue, it seems clear what is the cause of thrombosis in patient with the factor V Leiden defect. However, this chapter explores many aspects of factor V behavior and shows that, under some assay conditions, cleavage at residue 506 does not appear all that important. So, both of these chapter illustrate the difficulty that researchers often have in assigning a mechanism to clinical observations.

Part III, Novel Approaches to Therapy, describes ongoing research to overcome the current limitations of replacement therapy. Currently, the standard of care for hemophilia is replacement of the missing factor by injection of purified protein. One chapter describes the use of high dose factor VIIa to stimulate thrombin generation by a mechanism independent of the usual physiology of blood coagulation. Another chapter describes construction of factor VIII molecules that are hybrids between human factor VIII and porcine factor VIII (which is also used as a therapy in humans). These chimeric factor VIII molecules show promise to avoid the inhibitor development that plagues the use of both products. Dr. Mannucci and colleagues describe how a different method of administering the currently used human product can possibly improve patient care. Also, part III include a chapter on gene therapy, which provides the hope for curing, as opposed to treating, hemophilia by supplying a patient with the gene for the missing protein.

Finally, in Part IV, Inhibitor Development in Hemophilia Patients, chapters examine ways to overcome the serious problems that arise when neutralizing antibodies develop in hemophilia patients. These chapters look at how exciting research into basic immunology is leading to therapies that may go beyond overcoming the effect of inhibitors and actually block or reverse the formation of inhibitors in patients. The chapters look at B-cell, T-cell, and costimulatory mediated mechanisms of blocking inhibitors. The mechanisms proposed in these chapters may be the basis for new design of therapies.

A synergy between basic research and medical care has resulted in a number of improvements in the care of people with hemophilia. It is hoped that this book will become a resource for the ongoing dialogue between basic researchers, who can attack problems that are of ongoing concern to physicians, and physicians, who understand from patient interactions what the important problems are that need to be solved.

My thanks to the members of my lab who assisted me with the final preparation of the book for publication: Jennifer Browning, Alexis Henry, Eva Olson, Diane Palmieri, Jay Shelton, and Jennifer Wemhoff.

Dougald M. Monroe, Ph.D.
School of Medicine
The University of North Carolina at Chapel Hill

ACKNOWLEDGMENTS

The editors wish to thank the following sources for their generous educational grants in support of the symposium.

AHF, Inc.
American Red Cross
Baxter Hyland Immuno
Bayer Corporation, Pharmaceutical Division
Biogen, Inc.
Centeon LLC
Cerus Corporation
Chiron Corp.
The Coalition for Hemophilia B, Inc.
COBE BCT, Inc.
Genetics Institute
Green Mountain Antibodies, Inc.
Hemophilia Health Services
Nabi™
National Heart, Lung, and Blood Institute*
Novo Nordisk A/S
Speywood Pharmaceuticals, Inc.
Transkaryotic Therapies

* This publication was made possible by Grant Number 1 R13 HL62346-01 from the National Heart, Lung, and Blood Institute. Its contents are solely the responsibility of the authors and do not necessarily reflect the official views of the NHLBI.

SPONSORS

Hemophilia Care: An International Symposium in Honor of Harold R. Roberts, M.D., was presented by the UNC-CH Center for Thrombosis and Hemostasis, the Harold R. Roberts, M.D., Comprehensive Hemophilia Diagnostic and Treatment Center and the Hemophilia Treatment Centers in Region IV North. It was sponsored by the School of Medicine of the University of North Carolina at Chapel Hill.

Contents

1
THE TRANSFUSION-TRANSMITTED VIRUSES IN BLOOD TRANSFUSION

Naomi L.C. Luban, M.D.[1]
Rima F. Jubran, M.D.[2]
[1]Department of Transfusion Medicine, [2]Department of Hematology/Oncology
Childrens Hospital, National Medical Center
111 Michigan Ave NW, Washington, DC 20010

INTRODUCTION: THE RISKS OF BLOOD TRANSFUSION

Over the past 15 years, issues concerning the safety of the blood supply have caused significant changes in both national blood policies and the methods used in blood collection and screening in the United States. More specifically, the discovery that Human Immunodeficiency Virus (HIV) could be transmitted by blood transfusion heightened public awareness and concern. Multiple layers of protection now exist to reduce the risk of transmission of infectious agents through the transfusion of blood and blood components[1]. First, the donor pool is entirely voluntary, eliminating those persons donating for monetary gain. Second, extensive donor education and history-based screening procedures have been implemented. Third, extensive laboratory testing is performed on each donation. Finally, call back procedures and confidential unit exclusion provide mechanisms for donors who donated under peer pressure and believe they may provide a risk to transfusion recipients to indicate that their blood may not be suitable for transfusion. These multiple tiers of screening and testing have made the blood supply the safest it has ever been. The major threats that remain are in the donation of blood by seronegative donors during an infectious window period prior to detectable seroconversion and/or in the transmission of a virus or agent unrecognized as pathogenic and for which no test or process exists to eliminate it.

Hemophilia Care in the New Millennium, edited by D. Monroe *et al.*
Kluwer Academic/Plenum Publishers, 2001

Today, there are nine tests to screen for infectious disease risks. Current screening of blood donors in the United States includes testing for hepatitis B (HBV) and C (HCV), HIV-1 and -2, human T-lymphotropic virus-I and -II, syphilis, and optionally cytomegalovirus (Table 1). The current estimates of the risk of transfusion-transmitted viral infections have been made possible through the Retroviral Epidemiology Donor Study (REDS). This multi-institutional study funded by the National Heart, Lung & Blood Institute has permitted estimates of infectious window periods of risk. Using data from 2.3 million allogeneic blood collections which passed all donor screening, the risk of transmission in the United States is as follows: HIV, one in 493,000; HTLV, one in 641,000; HCV, one in 103,000; and HBV, one in 63,000[2]. With addition of p24 testing, HIV risk has been further returned to 1:676,000. There are sources of remaining risk to the blood supply. These may include an infectious but seronegative donor or one who has an immunosilent infection. Absence of a screening test or presence of a variant of a known agent that is not identified by the test methodology that is used is also a source of concern. Lastly, there can be laboratory error in the testing, labeling, quarantine and release of blood/blood products. Surveillance of donor and recipient pairs will permit identification of these rare sources of remaining risk but such surveillance programs are not well established in the U.S. except for individuals with clotting factor deficiencies and a soon to be implemented donor/recipient study in the REDS study.

In this chapter we will review some of the common transfusion-transmitted viral diseases with an emphasis on the limited donor and recipient exposure. Those individuals who receive pooled plasma products have the disadvantages of being exposed to extraordinary numbers of donors because of the manufacturing of these products; however these products undergo extensive processing methods like pasteurization, heat and solvent-detergent treatment which decrease viral infectivity. These topics will be covered by other authors in this symposium.

Newer assays that measure viral antigen rather than antibody response are being promulgated to identify donors who are infected prior to developing an antibody response. HIV p24 antigen testing, for example, was added in 1996 to decrease the risk of transfusion-transmitted HIV during the window period. The addition of HIV p24 antigen testing has reduced the window period to 6 days from about 16 days[3]. The risk of HIV has been recalculated to 1:641,000. The addition of similar assays in the future may decrease further the unwitting inclusion of infected donors in the blood supply. Molecular assays for more than one organism based on viral nuclear proteins using multiplex polymerase chain reaction (PCR) are now undergoing feasibility testing by the American Red Cross (ARC) and other blood suppliers. The goal of nucleic acid testing (NAT) of donors is to further exclude individuals who may be asymptomatic and viremic, but seronegative for HIV and HCV. Risk reduction will vary depending on the characteristics of the virus to be tested. Tests for additional viruses can be added as necessary. ARC estimates that NAT testing will identify per year 1/20,000 to 1/1,000,000 donors with HCV or between 40 and 300 immunosilent donors and anywhere from none to 5 HIV infected, immunosilent donors. They estimated a decrease in the HIV viremic window from 12-16 to 9-13 days and for HCV, a decrease in the HCV viremic period from 70 to 30 days. Preliminary studies in Europe have suggested that PCR (NAT) testing is both feasible and efficacious.

Table 1. Current blood donor screening

- Donor history and physical examination with attention to:
    - Physical stigmata suggesting alcohol use and parenteral drug use
    - History of a sexually transmitted disease, receipt of blood, blood products or derivatives, human tissue, dura mater, human growth hormone
    - History of donor or relative with Cruetzfeld-Jakob disease
    - History of viral hepatitis, malaria, babesiosis, Chagas disease
    - Sexual contact, incarceration, residing in household with individual with hepatitis B, HIV, or at risk for HIV
    - Specific questions for African birth, residence or travel with attention to eight specific areas with risk for HIV-type O
- Donor education and "warning literature"
- Informed consent
- Unit exclusion providing donor opportunity to request that unit not be used for transfusion
- Tests intended to prevent disease transmission
    - HBsAg
    - anti-HBc
    - anti-HTLV I/II
    - anti-HCV
    - anti-HIV-1/2
    - HIV-1 ag (p24)
    - Serologic test for syphilis

Optional: ALT and CMV

HUMAN IMMUNODEFICIENCY VIRUS

When it was discovered in late 1982 that HIV infection could be transmitted by blood and blood products, the Public Health Service recommended that persons at increased risk for HIV infection should not donate blood. In addition, blood collection centers began to implement safety measures such as the administration of high-risk behavior questionnaires and allowing donors the opportunity to exclude their blood after donation. The initiation of HIV antibody testing in 1985 resulted in a further decrease in transfusion-associated HIV infections. Only about 5 cases per year were reported to the Centers for Disease Control during the 5 years following implementation as compared with the 714 cases reported in 1984[4]. A test for antibodies to HIV type 2 was added, but it has had a small effect in the US, since only 3 donors out of 74 million tested were positive. In late 1995, HIV p24 antigen testing was added to further decrease the risk of transmitting HIV by shortening the window period. This has also had limited effects because the risk of HIV transmission is already very small. After screening 6 million donations, only 2 p24 antigen positive, HIV antibody negative donors have been identified[5].

Several studies have demonstrated that transfusion recipients have mortality rates that preclude their living long enough to develop a transfusion-transmitted disease. Pediatric patients are an exception. While ten year mortality rates of 52% are reported in adults[6], studies by our group have demonstrated long term survival of 83% in transfusion recipients[7]. They are a population in whom long-term adverse outcomes are more appropriately studied.

Two studies have reported on large numbers of children infected with HIV by transfusion. Jones *et al.* have published on 212 cases reported to the Centers for Disease Control from 1981 to 1987[8]. The mean age at HIV diagnosis was 4 years, with a range of 0.3 to 12.8 years. The median survival was 13.7 months, longer than the reported adult survival of 5.6 months.

Another study performed a retrospective look-back investigation of children transfused as neonates in an urban area with a high-risk donor population. They identified 33 HIV antibody positive children who were not previously diagnosed; of these, 13 were asymptomatic an average of 63 months following their transfusion[9]. Our own studies have reported children presenting symptom free as long as 9.5 years post transfusion. Parents of adolescents and preadolescents who present with HIV positive tests should be questioned about neonatal transfusions as a part of their HIV risk assessment.

HEPATITIS B VIRUS

HBV can be transmitted by cellular and noncellular blood and blood products. The implementation of third generation screening tests for hepatitis B surface antigen in 1975 caused a significant reduction in transfusion-transmitted HBV infection. HBV accounts for less than 10% of post-transfusion hepatitis[10]. Further reduction in the rates of hepatitis B and non A, non B hepatitis occurred when surrogate markers of hepatitis were introduced. Alanine aminotransferase as a reflection of acute hepatic inflammation and hepatitis B antibody, a marker of past HBV exposure were introduced in 1986.

Despite these specific and surrogate tests, hepatitis B remains a common transfusion transmitted virus. Acute disease develops in approximately 35% of persons infected with the virus and chronic infections occur in 1% to 10% of patients[11]. Chronically infected persons are at increased risk for developing chronic liver disease, cirrhosis and primary hepatocellular carcinoma later in life. The mechanism of hepatogenesis is not known, but an essential element may be the integration of the viral DNA into the host liver cell chromosome leading to either activation or suppression of cellular genes.

Treatment of HBV infection is primarily palliative and is aimed at providing symptomatic relief. In 1992, the Food and Drug Administration approved the use of interferon alpha-2b for the treatment of HBV and recent adult studies have shown promise. Forty to 50% of patients respond to treatment, but approximately half of them recur when treatment is stopped[12]. There is little experience in the use of interferon alpha in children, but the results are comparable with those for adults[13].

While investigations into treatment modalities for acquired HBV are ongoing, prevention remains the most important therapy. Immunization with recombinant HBV vaccine has been shown to decrease the seropositivity rate of acute HBV infection and the incidence of hepatocellular carcinoma in susceptible populations. Vaccination is recommended for all individuals with anticipated exposure to blood or blood products, and pre-vaccination testing is recommended for patients who have already received infusions of these products.

HEPATITIS A VIRUS

Hepatitis A virus is primarily spread in a fecal-oral manner via contaminated food or water. It is classically an acute self-limited illness with jaundice, fever, anorexia and malaise. Transmission by blood or blood product transfusion is rare, however there have been case reports of HAV infection due to contaminated solvent-detergent treated Factor VIII and Factor IX products in Europe and the United States[14-16]. The transmission of HAV by transfusion has been estimated to occur at a rate of 1 per 1 million units[11]. In accord with the US Advisory Committee on Immunization Practices, it is now recommended that all susceptible individuals who receive treatment with plasma-derived clotting factor concentrates also receive hepatitis A vaccine. There is no current treatment for HAV infection, however post-exposure prophylaxis with immune globulin is still recommended.

TRANSFUSION-TRANSMITTED VIRUS

Transfusion-Transmitted Virus (TTV) was recently identified by a Japanese laboratory from a patient with post-transfusion hepatitis. The viral genome consists of single-stranded, linear DNA of approximately 4 Kilobases and has no similarities at the genomic or amino acid level to any known virus family[17]. Although originally isolated from a patient with post-transfusion hepatitis, little is known of the pathophysiology of this virus, including routes of acquisition and association with disease. Viremia has been reported in 8-12% of blood donors in Japan, the United States, United Kingdom and Vietnam[17-19]. However, current PCR amplification techniques are not optimized to detect all TTV variants and more sensitive primers will likely reveal higher prevalence rates. Simmonds et al studied the prevalence of TTV in blood products and their recipients in the United Kingdom[18]. They found a prevalence rate of 1.9% in eligible blood donors. In addition TTV was detected frequently in recipients of non-virally inactivated factor VIII and IX concentrates prepared before 1986, but viral inactivation procedures reduced the frequency of detection from 9/12 (untreated) to 8/22 (treated). Their data suggested that inactivation of TTV in plasma pools by pasteurization at 60°C for 10 hours was more effective than solvent/detergent treatment, however larger studies are required to confirm this.

In a preliminary study, we found a prevalence rate of 65% (36/55) in healthy previously non-transfused children in the Washington, DC metropolitan area[20]. This high prevalence rate, as well as the presence of TTV in fecal samples of some patients, suggests that there may be more than one route of exposure.

In the original study of Nishizawa et al[17] TTV was implicated in post-transfusion hepatitis. However, subsequent studies have shown that while TTV may be transfusion-transmitted, the majority of infected individuals are asymptomatic with normal liver transaminases and minor to no changes in liver histology. Thus, TTV seems to be similar to Hepatitis G Virus exhibiting a high prevalence in the general population but with no clear association with disease at this time.

HEPATITIS C VIRUS

Hepatitis C virus is a single-stranded RNA virus belonging to the Flaviviridae family. The most common risk factors associated with HCV transmission in the United States include blood transfusion, injecting-drug use, and exposure to multiple sex partners. Studies have found that prior to implementing HCV screening 90% of post-transfusion non-A non-B hepatitis was caused by HCV[21]. However, HCV now is rarely transmitted by blood transfusion. First generation screening tests for HCV were developed and put into use in the spring of 1990 and targeted the c100-3 antigen. The use of second generation screening assays began in 1992 and were directed toward multiple epitopes: the c100-3 antigen, the core protein designated c22-3, and an NS3 protein designated c33c. Antibodies to the later two epitopes appear earlier than anti-c100-3. Eighty percent of HCV-infected individuals will develop specific antibody by 15 weeks from exposure and 100% by 6 months[21-22]. In the majority of individuals, anti-HCV antibodies persist for very long periods. Since the licensing of second-generation assays, the incidence of transfusion-acquired hepatitis has declined from 5% in 1989 to less than 1% and the risk of HCV infection has now been reduced to 1 in 103,000 transfusions[2].

Persons receiving clotting factor concentrates prepared from plasma pools were at very high risk for HCV infection until inactivation procedures were introduced in 1985 for Factor VIII, and 1987 for Factor IX. Hemophiliacs who were treated with products before that time have prevalence rates of HCV infection as high as 90%. In addition, since 1994, all immune globulin products have undergone inactivation procedures to ensure that they are negative for HVC RNA before release.

Acute post-transfusion hepatitis C infection is, in the majority of patients, asypmtomatic and anicteric. The significance of infection with HCV lies in the virus's propensity for persistent indolent infection. The mechanism of persistence is likely due to the ability of the virus to mutate rapidly under immune pressure and coexist as multiple mutants. These mutants have been termed quasi-species and they provide a mechanism for the virus to escape the immune response[22]. In addition, HCV can persist in the liver in a dormant state by down-regulating its replication to protect itself from immune clearance. Although there is an adequate humoral response to HCV, the antibodies rapidly become ineffective against emerging strains.

In both community-acquired and transfusion-associated HCV, the frequency of chronic hepatitis exceeds 60% and the frequency of persistent infection may exceed 90%. Of those with chronic hepatitis, two thirds will develop chronic active hepatitis, cirrhosis, or hepatocellular carcinoma (HCC). At least 20% of HCV infected patients will develop cirrhosis within two decades, and the risk for development of HCC is 1% to 5% after 20 years. The combined mortality from cirrhosis and HCC is 14.5% over a period ranging from 21 to 28 years[22]. Patients with chronic HCV hepatitis also can present with a variety of extrahepatic manifestations though to be of immunologic origin, such as arthritis, lichen planus, glomerulonephritis, keratoconjunctivitis sicca, and mixed cryoglobulinemia.

The majority of data concerning HCV infection in children comes from studies on multiple-transfused hematology and oncology patients diagnosed prior to the implementation of HCV screening. In children treated for malignancy, the prevalence of HCV varies between 17% and 40% depending on the geographic area[23-24]. Cesaro et al[24] found 117 HCV-positive patients of a total of 658 children who completed treatment for pediatric malignancy. Among the 117 patients, 91 (77.8%) had received at least one blood transfusion and chronic liver disease was found in 92 (78.6%). Fifty-one patients underwent liver biopsy and 1 out of 37 (2.7%) HCV positive only patients had cirrhosis as compared with 3 out of 14 (21.5%) HBV-HCV co-infected patients. No hepatic failure or hepatocellular carcinoma was noted after a 14-year follow-up period of these patients.

Because of the chronicity of HCV and the presumption that most recipients of blood from HCV antibody positive donors become infected, targeted look back programs have been implemented world-wide. The aim is to identify transfusion recipients who received blood from donors who later tested positive for HCV[25]. Canada and Denmark have reported on their initial programs which highlight what we can anticipate in the U.S. These include:

- 43% of identified patients had a congenital coagulopathy, chronic anemia, or malignancy.
- 26% of identified patients had blood during cardiovascular surgery.
- Most identified patients had received their transfusions between 1986 and 1991.
- 11% of subjects who underwent biopsy had histological cirihosis.
- The frequency of cirrihosis was higher in recipients who were infected after age 40[26-27].

Current treatment of adults with HCV infection consists of interferon alfa-2b, 2 million units 3 times weekly for 6 to 12 months. The sustained biochemical remission rate is approximately 20%, as about 50% of initial responders relapse after cessation of treatment[28]. As for acute-phase treatment, studies are underway to test the efficacy of single or combination drugs, including ribavirin and interferon and different interferons alone or in combinations. There is limited published experience on the use of interferon in children[29]. Given that HCV is a chronic disease with significant morbidity and mortality, early intervention has significant appeal, particularly in children. Look-back studies should, therefore target neonatal and pediatric transfusion recipients with consideration of therapy early in the child's clinical course.

HUMAN T-LYMPHOTROPIC VIRUSES I AND II

Human T-lymphotropic virus (HTLV)-I is a human retrovirus which is endemic in Japan, Sub-Saharan Africa, the Caribbean, Brazil, Melanesia, and Iran. HTLV-II is seen in endemic foci in native Indian populations in Panama, Brazil, Central Africa, and the United States. HTLV has been linked to T-cell leukemias, myelopathy, arthritis, and polymyositis. The first human retrovirus was isolated in 1978 from an individual with acute T cell leukemia. Subsequently, HTLV-I and -II have been characterized as oncoviruses that incorporate into the host DNA resulting in a life-long carrier state. Transmission occurs through transfusion, sexual contact, injection-drug use, and mother to infant in the peripartum period. The main cell involved in transmission is the lymphocyte.

Although infrequently reported, transfusion of HTLV-I and -II-infected cellular components has occured[30]. Blood that has been stored for more than 14 days and noncellular blood products do not appear to be infectious. Infection will develop in 20% to 60% of recipients of blood infected with HTLV-I or –II[31-32]. Transfusion-transmitted HTLV-I resulted in HTLV-I-associated myelopathy/ tropical spastic paraparesis in 4% to 8% of individuals, and in some patients an accelerated rate with progression of the neurologic disorder occurring within 1 month to 4 years after transfusion. To date, one case of T cell leukemia has been reported following transfusion of infected blood.

Donor screening for HTLV-I was introduced in 1988 through first-generation enzyme-linked immunoassay antibody test. Currently, HTLV-I and -II antibody tests are in use in the United States. Following screening with first-generation tests, the window period infection rate was estimated at 1 per 50,000 per unit[30], whereas in the REDS study, using second-generation assays, the rate was 1 in 641,000, the lowest rate of any transfusion-transmitted virus[2].

HEPATITIS G VIRUS/GBV-C VIRUS

Two independent groups of investigators discovered the RNA virus Hepatitis G, HGV, and its strain variant GBV-C. HGV belongs to the family Flaviviridae and has a 29% amino acid homology with HCV[33]. HGV is transmitted by parenteral routes including transfusion of blood and blood products, and is found in 1 to 2% of eligible volunteer blood donors in the United States[34]. Studies from different countries show similar prevalence rates, with the exception of Vietnam, where HGV was detected in 5.7% of healthy persons[35].

Currently, HGV can be detected by RNA polymerase reaction[36] and by an antibody to the envelope region E2 of the virus[37]. Anti-E2 is a recovery phase antibody that is usually detectable only after HGV RNA has been cleared. Studies have shown that the exposure rate among volunteer blood donors is 3 to 6 times the rate of viremia determined by identifying viral RNA. In high-risk groups such as hemophiliacs and injecting-drug users, the rates of exposure can be as high as 80% to 90% with viremia rates of 15 to 20%[38]. This large difference between exposure rates and active infection rates suggests that most of the HGV carriers eventually clear the virus. In one German study of intravenous drug users[39], HGV RNA significantly decreased over time from first injection drug use as opposed to HCV RNA that increased over time. This discrepancy between HGV and HCV may be due to the development of HGV-protective antibodies or other immune-mediated clearance mechanisms. Studies also show that among HCV-infected individuals, 10 to 20% are co-infected with HGV, however HGV had no effect on the clinical course of HCV infection or response to interferon therapy[38].

Although the virus can be transmitted by blood or blood product transfusion, there is no evidence that it is hepatotropic, nor has it been associated with a disease. Currently, there is no approved screening test for HGV, and no evidence that such a test would provide any benefit.

BACTERIAL CONTAMINATION

While transfusions are safer today than they have ever been, issues remain. Bacterial contamination of both red blood cells and platelets are far more common that viral disease transmission. Bacteria in platelet concentrates particularly, increase over time due to their room temperature storage. The risk of symptomatic complications or sepsis ranges from 1:2000 to 1:12000 transfusions. These estimates are 50 to 250 times greater than the risks for TTV.

Often the clinical presentation in the recipient is masked by the underlying condition of the patient. Mortality rates are very high: estimated to be 150 cases per year in the U.S. from gram negative platelet concentrate contamination alone[40]. Methods to rapidly detect bacterial contamination or to remove bacteria have been investigated without uniform acceptability, due to the lack of specificity and sensitivity of many of the assays. Sterilization of blood products using psoralen and long wavelength UV radiation has been shown to reduce growth of E coli, Saureos, and some bateriophage and animal viruses[41]. Recently the use of gamma radiation at doses as high as 7500 cGy was found to be ineffective in sterilizing platelet concentrates[42].

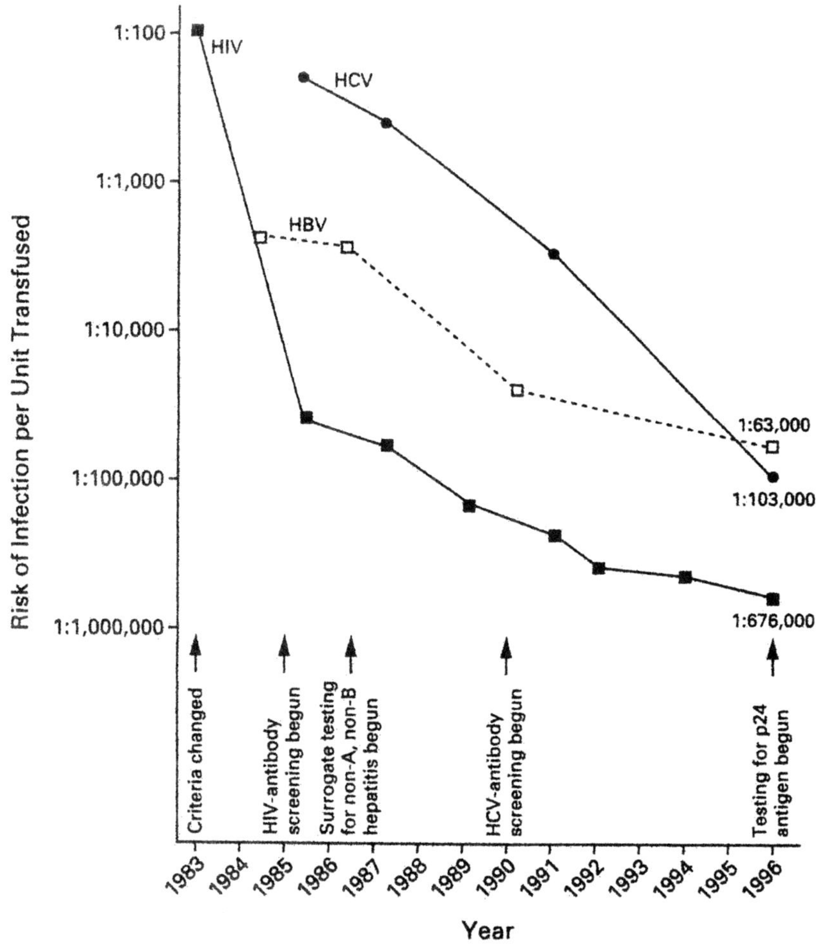

Figure 1. The Risks of Transfusion-Related Transmission of Human Immunodeficiency Virus (HIV), Hepatitis B Virus (HBV), and Hepatitis C Virus (HCV) in the United States. Each unit represents exposure to one donor. The risk of each of these infections has declined dramatically since 1983, the year the criteria for donor screening were changed; at that time the prevalence of HIV infection among donors was approximately 1 percent. Further declines have resulted from the implementation of testing of donor blood for antibodies to HIV beginning in 1985; surrogate testing for non-A, non-B hepatitis beginning in 1985-1987; testing for antibodies to HCV beginning in 1990; and testing for HIV p24 antigen beginning in late 1995. Reprinted with permission from L.T. Goodnough et al., "Transfusion Medicine. First of Two Parts – Blood Transfusion," New England Journal of Medicine 340(6):438-47, 1999 Feb 11.

CONCLUSION

In the future, we can expect the use of methodologies to process blood post collection to render them virologically and bacterially safe. It is unlikely, however, that pre-donation screening and testing will be dramatically modified until these post-collection processes are proven to be as, or more, efficacious than our current methods. New transfusion challenges like new variant Cruetzfeld-Jacob disease and other transfusion transmitted agents will continue to require our diligence in an effort to balance the potential decrease in the donor pool blood availability and avoidance of transfusion with patient need.

REFERENCES

1-Williams AE, Thomson RA, Schreiber GB et al. Estimates of infectious disease risk factors in US blood donors. JAMA 1997;277(12):967-972.

2-Schreiber GB, Busch MP, Kleinman SH et al. The risk of transfusion-transmitted viral infections. N Eng J Med 1996; 334(26):1685-1690.

3-Lackritz EM, Satten GA, Aberle-Grasse J et al. Estimated risk of transmission of the human immunodeficiency virus by screened blood in the United States. N Engl J Med 1995; 333:1721-5.

4-Roth WK, Weber M, Seifried E. Feasibility and efficacy of routine PCR screening of blood donations for hepatitis C virus, hepatitis B virus and HIV-1in a blood bank setting. Lancet 1999; 353:359-63.

5-Stamer SL, Aberle-Grasse J, Brodsky JP et al. US blood donor screening with p24 antigen (Ag): one year experience. Transfusion 1997;37:Suppl:1S.abstract.

6-Vamvakas E C, Taswell H F Long term survival after blood transfusion. Transfusion 1994; 34:471-7.

7-Wayne C, Cornell, M, O'Donnell R, Caldwell, B, Luban, N L. Seroprevalence of HIV in a transfused pediatric cardiac cohort in a high prevalence area. Transfusion 1993; 33:544

8-Jones DS, Byers RH, Bush TJ et al. Epidemiology of transfusion-associated acquired immunodeficiency syndrome in children in the United States, 1981 through 1989. Pediatrics 1993; 89:123-127.

9-Lieb L E, Mundy T M, Goldfinger D et al Unrecognized human immuno deficiency virus type 1 infection in a cohort of transfused neonates: a retrospective investigation. Pediatrics 1995; 95: 717-721.

10-Domen RE. Paid-versus-volunteer blood donation in the United States: A historical review. Transfus Med Rev 1995; 9:53-59.

11-Dodd RY. Adverse consequences of blood transfusion:Quantitative risk estimates. In Nance ST, ed. Blood supply:risks, perceptions, and prospects for the future. Bethesda, MD: American Association of Blood Banks 1994:1-24.

12-Carreno V, Castillo I, Molina J et al. Long-term follow-up of hepatitis B chronic carriers who responded to interferon therapy. J Hepatol 1992;15:102-106.

13-Lee WM. Hepatitis B Virus infection. N Eng J Med 1997;337(24):1733-1745.

14-Soucie JM, Robertson BH, Bell BP et al. Hepatitis A Virus infections associated with clotting factor concentrate in the United States. Transfusion 1998;38:573-579.

15-Manucci PM, Gdovin S, Gringeri A et al. Transmission of hepatitis A to patients with hemophilia by factor VIII concentrates treated with organic solvent and detergent to inactivate viruses. Ann Intern Med 1994;102:1-7.

16-Lawlor E, Johnson Z, Thornton L et al. Investigation of an outbreak of hepatitis A in Irish haemophilia A patients. Vox Sang 1994;67(suppl 1):18-20.

17-Nishizawa T, Okamoto H, Konishi K et al. A novel DNA virus (TTV) associated with elevated transaminase levels in posttransfusion hepatitis of unknown etiology. Biochem Biophys Res Commun 1997;241:92-97.

18-Simmonds P, Davidson F, Lycett C et al. Detection of a novel DNA virus (TT virus) in blood donors and blood products. Lancet 1998;352:191-195.

19-Naoumov NV, Petrova EP, Thomas MG et al. Presence of a newly described human DNA virus (TTV) in patients with liver disease. Lancet 1998;352:195-197.
20-Jubran RF, Dickstein B, Buu, M, et al. TTV viremia is common in healthy American and Vietnamese children. Presented at Pediatric Academic Society's Annual Meeting May 1-4, 1999, San Francisco.
21-Alter HJ. Transfusion transmitted Non-A, Non-B and Hepatitis C Infections in Principles of Transfusion Medicine, Rossi EC, ed. Baltimore, MD: Williams and Wilkins, 1996.
22-Alter HJ. To C or Not to C: these are the questions. Blood 1995;85:1681-1695.
23-Monteleone PM, Andrzejewski C, Keller JF. Prevalence of antibodies to hepatitis C virus in transfused children with cancer. Am J Pediatr Hematol Oncol 1994;16:309-313.
24-Cesaro S, Petris MG, Rossetti F et al. Chronic hepatitis C infection after treatment for pediatric malignancy. Blood 1997;90:1315-1320.
25-CDC. Recommendations for Prevention and Control of Hepatitis C virus (HCV) infection and HCV related chronic disease. MMWR Morb Mortal Wkly Rep 1998; 47: 1-39.
26-Christensen PB, Groenbaek K, Krarup HB et al Transfusion acquired hepatitis C:The Danish look back experience. Transfusion 1999; 39:188-193.
27-Larry A, Spurll G, Demers H, Goldman, M. Targeted hepatitis C look back, Quebec, Canada. Transfusion 1999: 39:194-200.
28-Management of hepatitis C:NIH consensus statement 1997, March 24-26;15(13), in press.
29-DiMarco V Lo Iacono O, Almasio P et al. Long-term efficacy of alpha I-interferon in B-thalassemics with chronic hepatitis C. Blood 1997;90:2207-2212.
30-Nelson KE, Donahue JG Munoz A et al . Transmission of retroviruses from seronegative donors by transfusion during cardiac surgery, a multicenter study of HIV-1 and HTLV-I/II infections. Ann Intern Med 1992;117:554-559.
31-Manns A, Wilks RJ, Murphy EL et al. A prospective study of transmission by transfusion of HTLV-1 and risk factors associated with seroconversion. Int J Cancer 1992;51:886-891.
32-Sullivan MT, Williams AE, Fang CT et al. Transmission of human T-lymphotopic virus types I and II by blood transfusion: retrospective study of recipients of blood components(1983 through 1988). the American Red Cross HTLV I/II Collaborative Study Group. Arch Intern Med 1991;151:2043-2048.
33-Linnen J, Wages J Jr, Zhang-Keck ZY et al. Molecular cloning and disease association of hepatitis G virus: a transfusion-transmissible agent. Science 1996;271:505-508.
34-Alter HJ, Nakatsuji Y, Melpoder J et al. The incidence of transfusion-associated hepatitis G infection and its relation to liver disease. N Eng J Med 1997;336:747-754.
35-Brown K, Wong S, Buu M et al. High prevalence of GB virus C/hepatitis G virus in healthy persons in Ho Chi Minh City, Vietnam. J Infec D 1997;175:450-453.
36-Schleuter V, Schmolke, M, Stark K et al. Reverse transcription-PCR detection of hepatitis G virus. J Clin Microbiol 1996;34:2660-2664.
37-Tacke M, Kiyosawa K, Stark et al. Detection of antibodies to a putative hepatitis G virus envelope protein. Lancet 1997;249:318-320.
38-Alter HJ. G-pers creepers, where'd you get those papers? A reassessment of the literature on hepatitis G virus. Transfusion 1997;37:569-572.
39-Stark K, Bienzle U, Hess G et al. Detection of the hepatitis G virus genome among injecting drug users, homosexual and bisexual men, and blood donors. J Infect Dis 1996;174:1320-1323.
40-Svaboda R, Lipton K S, Bacterial contamination of blood products American Association of Blood Banks Bulletin #96-6. AABB News Briefs 1996: 19(9): 10-11.
41-Lin L, Cook D N, Wiesenhahn G P et al. Photochemical inactivating viruses and bacteria in platelet concentrates by use of a novel psoralen and long wavelength ultraviolet light. Transfusion 1997; 37: 423-35.
42- Huston B M, Brecker M E, Bandarenks N. Lack of efficacy for conventional gamma irradiation of platelet concentrates to abrogate bacterial growth. Am J Clin Pathol. 1998; 109:743-747.
43-Goonough LT, Brecher ME, Kantor MH, Aubuchon, JP. Medical progress, Transfusion Medicine: Blood Transfusion. N. Engl. J. Med 1999; 340:438-447.

2

ARE PATIENTS WITH GLANZMANN THROMBASTHENIA AND THE BERNARD-SOULIER SYNDROME PROTECTED AGAINST ATHEROSCLEROSIS?

Alan T. Nurden[1], Paquita Nurden[2] and James N. George[3]

[1,2]Laboratoire de Pathologie Cellulaire de l'Hémostase, UMR 5533 CNRS, Hôpital Cardiologique, Pessac, France ; [3]Department of Medicine, Hematology-Oncology Section, University of Oklahoma Health Sciences Center, Oklahoma City, OK

Genetic defects of platelets give rise to bleeding syndromes of varying severity. Affected areas of platelet function include: the glycoprotein (GP) effectors of adhesion and aggregation, primary receptors for agonists, signalling pathways whereby messages are transmitted to targets elsewhere in the membrane or within the platelet, secretion from dense and α-granules, and the expression of procoagulant activity. *Glanzmann thrombasthenia (GT)* and the *Bernard-Soulier syndrome (BSS)* are the best characterized platelet diseases (1,2). GT is caused by abnormalities of platelet membrane GP IIb-IIIa (integrin $\alpha_{IIb}\beta_3$), resulting in absent platelet aggregation. BSS is caused by abnormalities of the GP Ib-V-IX complex, resulting in a loss of platelet adherence to vessel wall subendothelium. The knowledge gained from studies on platelet disorders has provided a better understanding of the

Hemophilia Care in the New Millennium, edited by D. Monroe *et al.*
Kluwer Academic/Plenum Publishers, 2001

molecular basis of primary hemostasis, and has helped in the development of new drugs for use in antithrombotic therapy. At the same time, the inability of platelets to bind to injured sites within the wall or to aggregate and form a thrombus in response to a haemostatic challenge raises the question as to whether such patients will be protected against atherosclerosis, for among the consequences of the altered platelet reactivity will be a decreased release of cytokines and growth factors potentially involved in atherosclerotic plaque development.

GLANZMANN THROMBASTHENIA

Defects primarily affecting surface components of platelets are shown in Fig. 1. Deficient platelet aggregation to all agonists is the hallmark of thrombasthenia. Ristocetin-induced binding of von Willebrand factor (vWF) to GT platelets is normal, however platelet 'agglutination' induced by ristocetin and vWF may occur in cycles. GT platelets bind to exposed subendothelial tissue. However, platelet spreading on the vessel wall surface and thrombus formation do not occur. Clot

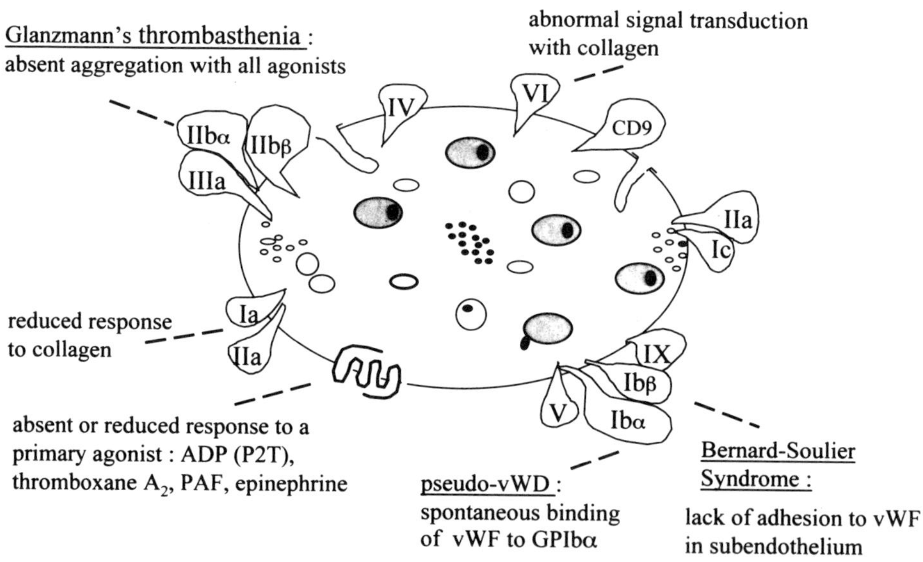

Figure 1. Cartoon showing the principal genetic disorders affecting glycoproteins of the surface membrane of platelets.

retraction is often defective. GP IIb-IIIa complexes physically mediate these processes. They also mediate 'outside-in' signalling, a phenomenon that occurs subsequent to the binding of fibrinogen and which may influence thrombus stability under normal conditions (3). The complexes also provide a link beween platelets and the coagulation system. Prothrombin can bind directly to GP IIb-IIIa, and this will not occur in thrombasthenia (4). Thrombasthenic platelets generate significantly less thrombin in response to tissue factor (5). Both fibrinogen and thrombin have known mitogenic effects on vascular cells.

Vitronectin receptor

The β_3 subunit in integrin nomenclature (GP IIIa) is also a component of the vitronectin receptor (VnR or $\alpha_V\beta_3$). In a normal situation, expression of the GP IIb gene (and therefore of GP IIb-IIIa complexes) is restricted to cells of the megakaryocytic lineage in man. However, VnR is found on endothelial cells, osteoclasts, fibroblasts, monocytes and activated B lymphocytes where it acts as a promiscuous receptor for adhesive protein ligands. This integrin is involved in angiogenesis, bone remodelling, tumour progression, implantation and placentation among other functions (6). VnR is a rare component in platelets, about 50 copies being found at the surface compared to 50,000 or more copies of GP IIb-IIIa (7). In GT, VnR is absent if the genetic lesion affects GP IIIa production (see below). Despite this, patients with β_3 gene defects do not have a more severe form of the disease. Initial results with β_3-integrin-deficient mice show normal vascularization, however, placental defects (and an increased mortality) and defective bone remodelling were seen (8). An initial evaluation in Israeli patients with GP IIb or GP IIIa gene defects was inconclusive as to whether additional defects were present when VnR was absent (9). If atherosclerosis is decreased in GT, then it would be logical that patients with GP IIIa gene defects are the most protected. Studies with transgenic mice should help here, particularly if cross-breeding leads to the production of α_{IIb} and β_3 deficiencies in strains already showing a genetically increased tendency for atherosclerosis.

Genetic defects

Although fibrinogen is the most frequently bound ligand for activated GP IIb-IIIa, vWF becomes important at high shear (10). That normal GP IIb-IIIa quaternary structure is required for its receptor activity is demonstrated by patients with variant forms of GT with qualitative defects of GP IIb-IIIa and absent fibrinogen receptor activity. However, most patients have little surface-expressed GP IIb-IIIa complex on their platelets and bleeding is a manifestation of this deficiency (2,11). The gene encoding GP IIb spans 17 kb and is comprised of 30 exons, that encoding GP IIIa spans 46 kb and is composed of 15 exons. The genes colocalize to 17q 21-23. Large gene deletions are rare, but splice defects, small insertions/deletions and point mutations are common (2,11).

Abnormalities within the GP IIb gene

In one of the first reports, Israeli Arab kindred were shown to possess a 13-bp deletion encompassing the splice acceptor site of exon 4 which resulted in alternative splicing to a downstream nucleotide AG receptor, producing a 6 aa deletion in the GP IIb protein (12). No surface GP IIb-IIIa was observed and the deleted sequence was shown to be critical for posttranslational processing of GP IIb. Defects leading to type I disease often involve the transmembrane domain of GP IIb. This is so in a French gypsy population (see 2,11). Sequence analysis of platelet RNA showed an 8-bp deletion at the 3' end of exon 15. This causes a frame shift leading to a premature stop codon and the synthesis of a severely truncated form of GP IIb. Several mutations within or near to Ca^{2+}-binding domains of GP IIb have been reported. GP IIb has four repeated 12 aa segments containing Asp and Glu residues and having a Ca^{2+}-binding function. Site-directed mutation and expression of recombinant glycoproteins in heterologous cell lines show that mutations in or near these domains inhibit transport of the complexes from the endoplasmic reticulum to the Golgi apparatus and/or export to the cell surface (reviewed in 2,11). In the absence of consanguinity, compound heterozygotes resulting from two defects within the GP IIb gene are a common cause of GT. In the case reported by Ruan et al (13), a maternal Glu_{324}->Lys mutation is associated with an Ile_{565}->Thr mutation on the father's allele. VnR may be present in about twice normal amounts in the platelets of patients with GP IIb gene defects (7).

Abnormalities within the GP IIIa gene

An early report concerned Iraqi Jews, where an 11 base deletion within exon 12 (now termed exon 13) resulted in a frame-shift and protein termination just before the transmembrane domain (12). This defect prevented normal membrane insertion of GP IIIa and expression of both GP IIb-IIIa and VnR. Several other splice site mutations or DNA deletions and inversions resulting in premature termination of GP IIIa have since been reported (see 2,11). A deletion/substitution ($Ile_{325}Pro_{326}Gly_{327}$ ->Met) in GP IIIa was reported (14). Expression of the mutated integrin in CHO cells showed that GP IIIa was synthesized but that VnR (the integrin studied) was not formed. Jin et al (15) reported a splice mutation associated with two different base changes which acted in concert and resulted in deletion of exon 9 and a 5-bp insertion which restored the reading frame. The result was a shorter GP IIIa unable to pair with GP IIb. Although the deletion was homozygous, consanguinity was denied and DNA microsatellite dinucleotide polymorphism analysis suggested the presence of two copies of the maternal chromosome. Mutations affecting cysteines have an important influence on GP IIIa structure and its capacity to complex with GP IIb. In one patient, a Cys_{374}->Tyr mutation resulted in only a 10 % expression of GP IIb-IIIa on the platelets (16). More GP IIb and GP IIIa were seen in Western blotting but proteolytic degradation of GP IIIa had occurred. The defect did not prevent complex formation but rather its stability or its transport to the surface. From our own work, a homozygous Cys_{542}->Arg mutation of the GP IIIa gene led to type I GT and a decreased VnR expression (17). Interestingly, this patient also suffers from tuberous sclerosis although there is no evidence to link the latter to the GP IIIa deficiency.

Variant Glanzmann thrombasthenia

In classic GT, GP IIb-IIIa complex formation does not occur or is severely reduced and the products of the functional gene (GP IIb or GP IIIa) are degraded intracellularly. In variants, the genetic defect generally affects fibrinogen receptor function rather than GP IIb-IIIa production. The patients are very heterogeneous and bleeding symptoms range from severe to mild. The first such report described an Asp_{119}->Tyr substitution within an RGD-binding site on GP IIIa and which forms part of the ligand-binding pocket (18). Three patients from unrelated families have GP IIb and GP IIIa subunits which dissociate more rapidly on Ca^{2+}-chelation. Studies on these patients have revealed that the codon for Arg_{214} of the GP IIIa gene is a mutational hotspot (reviewed in 2,11). The affected sequence is critical for maintaining the correct conformation of the GP IIb-IIIa complex and its modification prevents the expression of the ligand-binding pocket in response to platelet stimulation.

Variant (R.P.) has about half the normal platelet GP IIb-IIIa content, and his platelets fail to bind fibrinogen when stimulated by ADP. A heterozygous Ser_{752}->Pro point mutation was detected in the cytoplasmic domain of GP IIIa (19). Studies on transfected CHO cells confirmed a role for the GP IIIa cytoplasmic domain in 'inside-out' signalling and expression of the extracellular ligand-binding epitopes of GP IIb-IIIa (see 3). A somewhat similar finding was reported for the variant described by Wang et al (20). Here, a heterozygous C2268T nucleotide substitution within exon 13 of the maternal allele of the GP IIIa gene resulted in a stop codon in place of Arg_{724} producing a truncated protein containing only the first eight of the 47 aa normally present in the cytoplasmic domain. Interestingly, in both of the above patients only the affected allele was expressed. Patient (A.P.) has a 'thrombasthenia-like' syndrome in that the platelet aggregation response was not null but was much reduced in velocity and intensity. Total platelet GP IIb-IIIa content was about 50% of normal, but the surface pool of GP IIb-IIIa was decreased to about 18%. These residual complexes were functional and their density may be at the threshold of the amount required to support platelet aggregation. A heterozygous Arg_{995}->Gln substitution in the GFFKR sequence of the cytoplasmic domain of GP IIb was detected and shown in transfection experiments to account for the reduced surface expression of the residual GP IIb-IIIa complexes in platelets (21). A more recent finding from our laboratory (ATN), has identified a Leu_{196}->Pro substitution in the extracellular domain of GP IIIa in a new GT variant (R.M.) also thought to be a compound heterozygote. The patient is a 70 year old man and his mother, also heterozygous for the above mutation but with a normal GP IIIa allele, is now 98 years old. Obligate heterozygotes for the classic form of GT have intermediate concentrations of GP IIb-IIIa and no bleeding syndrome. The findings from the Bordeaux family at least prove the potential for longevity in the presence of an abnormal β_3 allele.

Other comments

Myocardial infarction and occlusive arterial thrombosis have not been reported in GT. However, this could be because the published case histories mostly concern young patients. This was highlighted in the review of the literature performed by George, et al. (22) who reported that the average age of 113 patients (58 % women) at the time of their initial report was about 20 years. Purpura, epistaxis, gingival haemorrhage and menorrhagia are the most common forms of bleeding in GT. Bleeding from large vessels is rare in the absence of trauma. Interestingly, there have been two reports of life-threatening venous thrombosis in GT patients. The first was in variant (R.P.) (see above), who developed proximal deep vein thrombosis after a long air flight (23). The second was patient (A.M.) reported by George, et al. (22). Now a middle-aged woman, this patient with type I disease (<5% GP IIb-IIIa) and a homozygous Cys_{457}->Tyr mutation in GP IIIa, suffered from a severe proximal deep vein thrombosis during adolescence. Well-characterized risk factors for venous thrombosis such as the Factor V Leiden or the 20210 G->A prothrombin gene polymorphism were studied in a series of 14 unrelated GT patients by Guyonnet Duperat, et al (24). Only one patient showed the Factor V Leiden abnormality and none the prothrombin polymorphism, showing that these two factors were unlikely to account for the wide variations in bleeding tendency seen among GT patients.

BERNARD-SOULIER SYNDROME

BSS is characterized by autosomal recessive inheritance, thrombocytopenia, decreased platelet survival in most patients, and giant platelets. Platelet counts range from as low as 20,000/μl to near normal. BSS is rarer than GT and this has been suggested to be due to the compactness of the genes and the lack of introns (25). The platelets on peripheral blood smears may be up to 20 μ in diameter. Electron microscopy showed a large number of cytoplasmic vacuoles and membrane complexes in the giant platelets and these abnormalities extended to megakaryocytes (MK) where an irregular appearance of the demarcation membrane system is a common feature (reviewed in 26). These changes in MK ultrastructure may contribute to the thrombocytopenia and the formation of large platelets.

Platelet function abnormalities

BSS platelets aggregate normally with agonists such as ADP and collagen, but fail to agglutinate when platelet-rich plasma (PRP) is stirred with ristocetin or botrocetin. The lack of binding of vWF to GP Ib accounts for this and the decreased adherence to subendothelium which characterizes BSS. Thus the functional defect is similar to that observed in von Willebrand disease. The interaction of vWF with elements of the subendothelium exposes epitopes reactive with GP Ib but which are inaccessible on freely circulating multimers. In normal primary hemostasis the initial attachment of platelets by way of the GP Ib/vWF axis is then stabilized by interactions involving GP IIb-IIIa and/or GP Ia-IIa (27). Aggregation of BSS platelets by thrombin is abnormal, with decreased thrombin binding, a prolonged lag phase and a reduced intensity. GP Ibα contains one or more high-affinity thrombin binding sites located within an anionic sulfated-tyrosine sequence in the N-terminal domain (28). The residual response of BSS platelets to thrombin is presumably mediated through the moderate-affinity receptors of the protease-activated receptor (PAR) family (PAR-1, PAR-3, PAR-4). Although little is known of PAR-3 and PAR-4 expression in BSS, platelets from such patients aggregate normally to thrombin-receptor activating peptide (TRAP) reactive with PAR-1 (29). Diminished coagulant activity was reported in early studies on BSS platelets although the mechanics of this remain to be elucidated.

Genetic defects in Bernard-Soulier syndrome

The products of four genes (Ibα, Ibβ, IX and V) assemble to form the GP Ib-IX-V complex (see 25). The genes for GP Ibα and GP Ibβ are on chromosomes 17 and 22, while those encoding GP IX and GP V are on chromosome 3. Each protein is a member of the leucine-rich motif superfamily, suggesting a common ancestral gene. Except for GP Ibβ, the coding sequence is contained within a single exon. The bulk of GP Ibα, Ibβ, IX and V form a complex with a stoichiometry of 2:2:2:1, thus the complex is large. Flow cytometry allows an evaluation of platelet size, while also permitting the assessment of GP Ib-IX-V levels (30). Obligate heterozygotes for the classic form of the disease have intermediate concentrations of GP Ib-IX-V. Although mild hemorrhagic episodes have been reported, most heterozygotes do not experience abnormal bleeding. GP Ibα has been reported to be synthesized by endothelial cells, indeed evidence has been obtained for the presence of the entire GP Ib-IX-V complex (31). However, there are no reports of an abnormal endothelial cell function in BSS.

Defects of the GP Ibα gene

These are the most frequently detected in BSS (see 25, for a complete list). Truncation of GP Ibα with loss of the transmembrane domain has been reported for several cases. An example comes from the work of Kunishima et al (32), who described a homozygous C->A substitution and a shortened GP Ibα stopping at Ser_{444}. The truncated molecule was secreted into the plasma. In another patient a homozygous single base pair mutation T->A leading to a Cys_{209}->Ser substitution was reported. Here, an abnormal folding of GP Ibα in the absence of disulfide formation prevented complex formation (33). The interactions responsible for the noncovalent heterodimer association of GP Ib, GP IX and GP V are still not known, but transfection studies have demonstrated that cDNAs for each of GP Ibα, GP Ibβ, and GP IX are required for cell surface expression of the proteins (data reviewed in 25). GP V is the only one of the four polypeptides that can be expressed alone in significant amounts on the surface of transfected cells.

Defects of the GP Ibβ and GP IX genes

Budarf et al (34) first showed that defects in the GP Ibβ gene may give rise to BSS. The patient was not a classic case, for as well as possessing giant platelets (and decreased ristocetin-induced platelet aggregation), he suffered from a developmental disorder, the DiGeorge/Velo-cardio-facial syndrome. The patient was in fact a compound heterozygote. The first abnormal allele resulted from a deletion in 22q11.2, the site of localization of the GP Ibβ gene, and a zone known to be affected in the DiGeorge syndrome (34). The second abnormality related to a single point mutation (C ->G) at -133 of the Ibβ gene, a site for the GATA-1 transcription factor (35). The first reported defect in the GP IX gene involved double heterozygosity: (a) an A->G transition in codon 21 resulted in an Asp->Gly conversion and (b) an A->G change in codon 45 converted Asn->Ser (36). These changes concerned conserved residues in or flanking the single leucine-rich glycoprotein motif of GP IX. A homozygous Asn_{45}->Ser substitution was subsequently reported (37). Other mutations within the leucine-rich repeat have since been described, as has a nonsense mutation in codon 126 resulting in a truncated protein without the transmembrane domain (data reviewed in 2,25).

Variant-type Bernard-Soulier syndrome

Here, qualitative defects lead to a nonfunctional GP Ib-IX-V complex that is at least partially expressed in platelets which remain giant. For the 'Bolzano' variant, platelets failed to bind some but not all monoclonal antibodies to GP Ibα, and immunoblotting confirmed the presence of GP Ibα and GP IX. The binding of thrombin to the patient's platelets was normal, yet the ability of GP Ibα to bind vWF had been lost (data reviewed in 2,25). A homozygous Ala_{156}->Val substitution in the sixth leucine-rich repeat of GP Ibα was shown to be responsible for this unique phenotype (38). As the principal vWF-binding domain of GP Ibα is contained within a disulfide-bonded double loop region subterminal to the leucine repeats (see 25), the Ala_{156} ->Val substitution may induce conformational changes that extend to and render nonfunctional the vWF-binding domain. Another variant was detected in a family with an autosomal dominant form of the disease and a Leu_{57}->Phe substitution within the first leucine-rich repeat (39). In variant Nancy I, a 3-bp deletion resulted in the loss of Leu_{179} in the seventh leucine-rich repeat of GP Ibα (40). Two patients have been reported where platelets show about 40 % of residual vWF binding but normal surface GP V and where the first leucine within the fifth leucine repeat sequence of GP Ibα was substituted by a Pro (see 2,25). Transient transfection experiments in mouse L-cells proved that the presence of Pro_{129} in GP Ibα was responsible for the patients' phenotype. The Karlstrad variant results from a Trp_{498}->Stop mutation leading to a truncated glycoprotein Ibα (see 2,25). In contrast to other truncated forms of GP Ibα (see above), this variant contains part of the transmembrane domain as well as the disulfide linking the Ibα and β subunits. Finally, Kunishima et al (41) reported a patient with a mild bleeding disorder and where most of the platelet GP Ibα was not disulfide-linked to GP Ibβ as a result of two missense mutations in the GP Ibβ gene.

Other comments

BSS is an extremely rare disease, 88 patients (47 women) were described in a recent review (25). Epistaxis, gingival and mucocutaneous bleeding are again the most common forms of bleeding (2). Hemorrhage is mostly associated with trauma. The fact that coronary artery atherosclerosis and unstable angina can occur in BSS is based on a single report of a patient who successfully underwent a bypass operation (42). However, as with GT, most patients are reported when at an early age. Transgenic mouse models for the GP Ibα, GP IX and GP V genes are beginning to be available for study and will help ascertain whether patients with BSS are protected against atherosclerosis.

It should be noted that platelet-type or pseudo-von Willebrand disease is also associated with an abnormality of the platelet GP Ib-IX-V complex. However, in this disease there is an unusual gain of function phenotype with abnormally increased binding of plasma vWF to platelets. The mutations giving rise to this disorder are Gly_{233}->Val and Met_{239}->Val (data reviewed in 2,25). These amino acid substitutions occur within the disufide-bonded double loop region of GP Ibα. The mutant GP Ibα binds normal human vWF multimers spontaneously, so that the latter are cleared from the plasma and the result is a clinical condition typical of von Willebrand disease.

OTHER INHERITED DISORDERS OF PLATELETS

Primary receptor deficiencies

A patient was reported with a mild, lifelong bleeding disorder where a selective absence of aggregation and adhesion to collagen was associated with a deficiency of GP Ia-IIa (43). GP Ia-IIa ($\alpha_2\beta_1$) is a platelet collagen receptor and a member of the integrin β_1 subfamily. Later, a patient deficient in GP VI was also shown to lack a collagen-induced aggregation response (44). The potential explanation is that the platelet/collagen interaction is mediated by platelets attaching through GP Ia-IIa in flowing blood and then becoming activated through a second receptor, GP VI, by a mechanism mimicked by convulxin A, a protein isolated from snake venom (45). So far, only isolated patients have been reported, although numbers may increase when appropriate testing procedures are introduced. Care must be taken with such patients to rule out changes in collagen receptor density due to intronic polymorphisms (46). Three α_2 gene alleles defined by eight polymorphisms are associated with a threefold difference in expression levels of GP Ia-IIa on platelets. The rate of platelet attachment to collagen in whole blood at high shear is proportional to receptor density (46). These polymorphisms can either (i) be a risk factor for thrombosis in arterial disease or (ii) define bleeding risk in von Willebrand disease (data reviewed in 47). Particularly interesting is the potential for similar density variations on vascular cells (endothelium, fibroblasts, smooth muscle cells) which express this integrin. If this is truly the case, then variations in atherosclerotic plaque growth and perhaps susceptibility for fissuring could be expected.

Current evidence suggests that there are at least 3 platelet receptors for ADP:$P2X_1$, an ion channel linked to Ca^{2+} influx; $P2Y_1$ thought to mediate ADP-induced Ca^{2+}-mobilization and shape change; and $P2T_{AC}$, responsible for macroscopic platelet aggregation and linked to adenylate cyclase (48). Two groups have reported patients with a hereditary disease linked to a much decreased platelet aggregation to ADP despite a normal shape change and Ca^{2+} -mobilisation (see 49,50). A much reduced binding of radiolabeled 2-MeS-ADP (a stable analogue of ADP) together with the specific inability of ADP to lower the cAMP content of PGE_1-stimulated platelets, suggests that the $P2T_{AC}$ receptor is affected. These patients show identical functional changes to normal platelets treated with the anti-platelet drugs, ticlopidine and clopidogrel. The synergistic role of ADP in the platelet response to low doses of other stimuli means that the platelets also show a decreased sensitivity to agonists such as thromboxane A_2 (TXA_2) (51). Elsewhere, an Arg_{60} -> Leu mutation has been identified in the TXA_2 receptor (52). Platelet pathologies may also concern the signal transduction pathways into which surface receptors are locked (Fig. 2). Such defects include an impaired Ca^{2+} mobilization, defective inositol-1,4,5-triphosphate ($InsP_3$) production and reduced phosphorylation of proteins by protein kinase C or tyrosine kinases (data reviewed in 1). Patients with congenital deficiencies of cyclooxygenase, thromboxane synthetase, lipoxygenase, glycogen-6 synthetase and of ATP metabolism have all been reported and lead to platelet function abnormalities often resembling those seen in storage pool disease (see Figure 2). Although nothing is known about possible protection from atherosclerosis in these disorders, they could provide useful information relevant to any possible protective effect afforded by long term therapy with clopidogrel (or ticlopidine) and/or aspirin.

Defects of secretion

Alpha granules are the storage site for proteins which may be synthesized in MK (e.g. platelet factor 4 [PF4], β-thromboglobulin [β-TG], vWF) or endocytosed from plasma (e.g. fibrinogen, albumin, immunoglobulin). Their membranes contain a

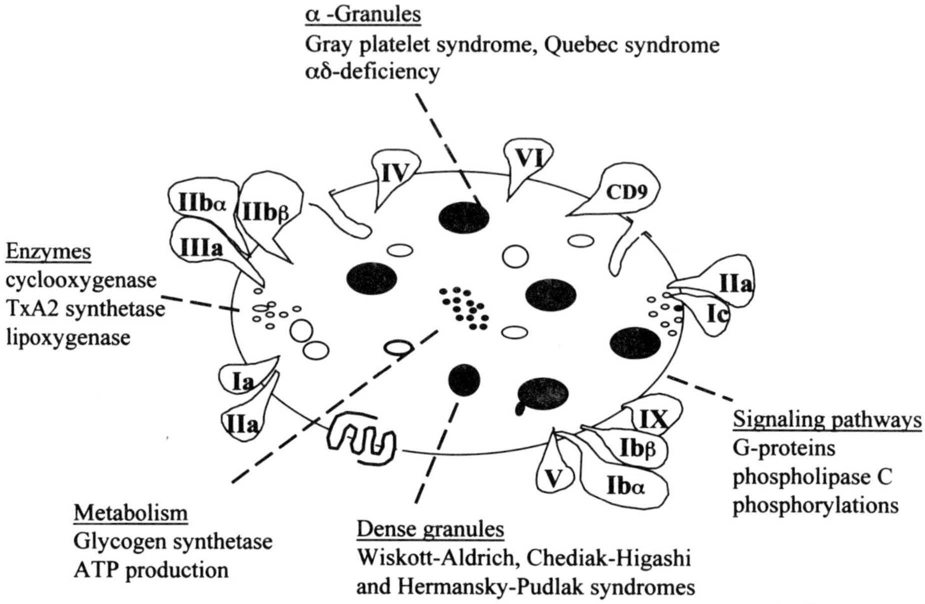

Figure 2. Cartoon showing the principal genetic disorders affecting intracellular sites in platelets.

variety of glycoproteins some of which are exclusive to the granule membrane in unactivated platelets, P-selectin being an example. Although secondary deficiencies of α-granule proteins may be associated with inherited disorders of plasma proteins or membrane glycoproteins (e.g factor V deficiency; fibrinogen in GT or afibrinogenemia; vWF in von Willebrand's disease), the primary defect may also concern the platelet α-granule. The Gray platelet syndrome (GPS) is a mild bleeding disorder with predominantly an autosomal recessive inheritance that is characterized by the platelet's inability to store α-granule proteins (see 1). As a result, secretion-dependent platelet aggregation can be abnormal. A feature of this disorder is the early onset of myelofibrosis, a finding attributed to the inability of MK to retain newly synthesized platelet-derived growth factors that are deposited directly within the marrow (53). GPS is the only inherited platelet disorder where the platelet defect leads to a so far proven pathological consequence on other cells. The Quebec platelet syndrome is an autosomal dominant bleeding disorder described in two French-Canadian families. Here, platelets have a severe multimerin deficiency and show protease-related degradation of many α-granule proteins (including P-selectin and factor V) even though α-granule ultrastructure is preserved (reviewed in 53).

Multimerin is a multimeric protein that is stored complexed with factor V in the α-granules. In αδ-Storage pool disease, the platelet deficiency extends to the contents of both dense and α-granules. Secretion-dependent platelet aggregation is more severely affected than in GPS and adhesion may also be reduced (data reviewed in 54). The molecular bases for the above-cited α-granule disorders have not yet been determined.

Dense (δ) granules are the storage sites for serotonin and nucleotides such as ADP and ATP. This type of deficiency may be quite common and should always be considered when a patient presents with a deficiency of secretion-dependent aggregation. The decreased platelet serotonin content means that vasoconstriction can be reduced at sites of platelet accumulation. Congenital defects of platelet dense granules also occurs in diseases affecting more than one type of cell such as the Wiskott-Aldrich, Hermansky-Pudlak and Chediak-Higashi syndromes (1,55). The latter two syndromes are rare autosomal recessive diseases in which a bleeding diathesis is accompanied by deficient pigmentation of the skin and hair (affecting melanosomes) and a defective lysosomal function in many cell types. In the Wiskott-Aldrich syndrome the defect extends primarily to the immune system. In each of these disorders the gene carrying the defect has been identified and shown to encode proteins involved in signalling and/or granule maturation (1,55).

Scott syndrome

Mention must be made of the Scott syndrome, a rare inherited disorder of Ca^{2+}-induced phospholipid scrambling and assembly of the prothombinase complex on blood cells including platelets (see 56). In brief, Scott platelets fail to transport phosphatidylserine (PS) from the inner to the outer phospholipid leaflet of the membrane bilayer, with the result that factors Va and Xa fail to bind leading to the incapacity of the activated cell surface to transform prothrombin to thrombin. This lack of thrombin generation is sufficient to induce a bleeding diathesis. As thrombin is a powerful mitogen in the vessel wall, patients with the Scott syndrome or related disorders are also likely candidates for possessing a protective effect against atherosclerosis.

FINAL COMMENTS

It is clear that the rareness of patients with inherited platelet disorders means that no firm conclusions can be made as to whether the patients are protected or not against atherosclerosis. In the future, the reproduction of human platelet disorders in mouse models of atherosclerosis may provide more definitive answers concerning the role of platelets in this highly important disease of the vessel wall. Meanwhile, the opening of a registry to assemble details of cardiovascular diseases in patients with inherited disorders of platelet function would be worthwhile.

REFERENCES

1. Nurden AT. Inherited abnormalities of platelets. Thromb Haemost, In press.

2. Nurden AT, George JN: Inherited disorders of the platelet membrane: Glanzmann thrombasthenia, Bernard-Soulier syndrome and other disorders. In Colman RW, Hirsh J, Marder VJ, Clowes AW, George JN (eds): Hemostasis and Thrombosis. Basic Principles and Clinical Practice. Vol IV. Philadelphia, JB Lippincott Co, In Press

3. Shattil SJ, Kashiwagi H, Pampori N: Integrin signalling: The platelet paradigm. Blood 1998; 91: 2645-57.

4. Byzova TV, Plow EF: Networking in the hemostatic system. Integrin $\alpha_{IIb}\beta_3$ binds prothrombin and influences its activation. J Biol Chem 1997; 272: 27183-8.

5. Reverter JC, Beguin S, Kessels H, Kumar R, Hemker HC, Coller BS: Inhibition of platelet-mediated, tissue factor-induced thrombin generation by the mouse/human chimeric 7E3 antibody. Potential implications for the effect of c7E3 Fab treatment on acute thrombosis and 'clinical restenosis'. J Clin Invest 1996; 98: 863-74.

6. Friedlander M, Brooks PC, Shaffer RW, Kincald CM, Varner JA, Cheresh DA: Definition of two angiogenic pathways by distinct α_v integrins. Science 1995; 270: 1500-2.

7. Coller BS, Cheresh DA, Asch E, Seligsohn U: Platelet vitronectin receptor expression differentiates Iraqi-Jewish from Arab patients with Glanzmann thrombasthenia in Israel. Blood 1991; 77: 75-83.

8. Hodivala-Dilke KM, McHugh KP, Tsakiris DA, Rayburn H, Crowley D, Ullman-Culleré M, Ross FP, Coller BS, Teitelbaum S, Hynes RO: β_3-integrin-deficient mice are a model for Glanzmann thrombasthenia showing placental defects and reduced survival. J Clin Invest 1999;103: 229-38.

9. Coller BS, Seligsohn U, Peretz H, Newman PJ: Glanzmann thrombasthenia: New insights from an historical perspective. Sem Hematol 1994; 31: 301-11

10. Goto S, Ikeda Y, Saldivar E, Ruggeri ZM: Distinct mechanisms of platelet aggregation as a consequence of different shearing flow conditions. J Clin Invest 1998; 101: 479-86.

11. French DL: The molecular genetics of Glanzmann's thrombasthenia. Platelets 1998; 9: 5-20.

12. Newman PJ, Seligsohn U, Lyman S, Coller BS: The molecular genetic basis of Glanzmann thrombasthenia in the Iraqi-Jewish and Arab populations in Israel. Proc Natl Acad Sci USA 1991; 88: 3160-4.

13. Ruan J, Peyruchaud O, Alberio L, Valles G, Clemetson K, Bourre F, Nurden AT: Double heterozygosity of the GP IIb gene in a Swiss patient with Glanzmann's thrombasthenia. Br J Haematol 1998; 102: 918-25.

14. Morel-Kopp M-C, Kaplan C, Proulle V, Jallu V, Melchior C, Peyruchaud O, Aurousseau M-H, Kieffer N: A three amino acid deletion in glycoprotein IIIa is responsible for type I Glanzmann's thrombasthenia: Importance of residues $Ile^{325}Pro^{326}Gly^{327}$ for β_3 integrin subunit association. Blood 1997; 90: 669-77.

15. Jin Y, Dietz HC, Montgomery RA, Bell WR, McIntosh I, Coller B, Bray PF: Glanzmann thrombasthenia. Cooperation between sequence variants in*Cis* during splice selection. J Clin Invest 1996; 98: 1745-54.

16. Grimaldi CM, Chen F, Scudder LE, Coller BS, French DL: A Cys374Tyr homozygous mutation of platelet glycoprotein IIIa (β_3) in a Chinese patient with Glanzmann's thrombasthenia. Blood 1996; 88: 1666-75.

17. Ruan J, Schmugge M, Clemetson KJ, Cazes E, Combrié R, Bourre F, Nurden AT: Homozygous Cys542->Arg mutation of the GP IIIa gene in a Swiss patient with type I Glanzmann's thrombasthenia. Br J Haematol 1999; 105: 523-531.

18. Loftus JC, O'Toole TE, Plow EF, Glass A, Frelinger AL III, Ginsberg MH: A β_3 integrin mutation abolishes ligand binding and alters divalent cation-dependent conformation. Science 1990; 249: 915-8.

19. Chen Y, Djaffar I, Pidard D, Steiner B, Cieutat AM, Caen JP, Rosa JP: Ser^{752}->Pro mutation in the cytoplasmic domain of integrin β_3 subunit and defective activation of platelet integrin $\alpha_{IIb}\beta_3$ (glycoprotein IIb-IIIa) in a variant of Glanzmann's thrombasthenia. Proc Natl Acad Sci USA 1992; 89: 10169-73.

20. Wang R, Shattil SJ, Ambruso DR, Newman PJ: Truncation of the cytoplasmic domain of β_3 in a variant form of Glanzmann thrombasthenia abrogates signaling through the integrin $\alpha_{IIb}\beta_3$ complex. J Clin Invest 1997; 100: 2393-403.

21. Peyruchaud O, Nurden AT, Milet S, Macchi L, Pannochia A, Bray PF, Kieffer N, Bourre F: R to Q aminoacid substitution in the GFFKR sequence of the cytoplasmic domain of the integrin α_{IIb} subunit in a patient with a Glanzmann's thrombasthenia-like syndrome. Blood 1998; 92: 4178-87.

22. George JN, Caen JP, Nurden AT: Glanzmann's thrombasthenia: The spectrum of clinical disease. Blood 1990; 75: 1383-95.

23. Gruel Y, Parcouret G, Bellucci S, Caen J: Severe proximal deep vein thrombosis in a Glanzmann thrombasthenia variant successfully treated with a low molecular weight heparin. Blood 1997; 90: 888-90.

24. Guyonnet Duperat V, Vergnes C, Nurden P, Nurden AT: Screening for Factor V Leiden and a prothrombin gene polymorphism in patients with Glanzmann's thrombasthenia. Br J Haematol 1998; 101: 592-6.

25. Lopez JA, Andrews RK, Afshar-Kharghan V, Berndt MC: Bernard-Soulier syndrome. Blood 1998; 91: 4397-418.

26. Nurden P, Nurden AT: Giant platelets, megakaryocytes and the expression of glycoprotein Ib-IX complexes. CR Acad Sci Paris 1996; 319: 717-26.

27. Savage B, Almus-Jacobs F, Ruggeri ZM: Specific synergy of multiple substrate-receptor interactions in platelet thrombus formation under flow. Cell 1998; 94: 657-66.

28. Mazzucato M, De Marco L, Masotti A, Pradella, P, Bahou WF, Ruggeri ZM: Characterization of the initial α-thrombin interaction with glycoprotein Ibα in relation to platelet activation. J Biol Chem 1998; 273: 1880-7.

29. Kahn ML, Zheng Y-W, Huang W, Bigornia V, Zeng D, Moff S, Farese RV Jr, Tam C, Coughlin SR: A dual thrombin receptor system for platelet activation. Nature 1998; 394: 690-4.

30. Tomer A, Scharf RE, McMillan R, Ruggeri ZM, Harker LA: Bernard-Soulier syndrome: quantitative characterization of megakaryocytes and platelets by flow cytometric and platelet kinetic measurements. Eur J Haematol 1994; 52: 193-200.

31. Wu G, Essex DW, Meloni FJ, Takafuta T, Fujimura K, Konkle BA, Shapiro SS: Human endothelial cells in culture and in vivo express on their surface all four components of the glycoprotein Ib/IX/V complex. Blood 1997; 90: 2660-9.

32. Kunishima S, Miura H, Fukutani H, Yoshida H, Osumi K, Kobayashi S, Ohno R, Naoe T: Bernard-Soulier syndrome Kagoshima: Ser444 ->stop mutation of glycoprotein (GP) Ibα resulting in circulating truncated GP Ibα and surface expression of GPIbβ and GPIX. Blood 1994; 84: 3356-62.

33. Simsek S, Noris P, Lozano M, Pico M, von dem Borne AEG, Ribera A, Gallardo D: Cys209Ser mutation in the platelet membrane glycoprotein Ibα gene is associated with Bernard-Soulier syndrome. Br J Haematol 1994; 88: 839-44.

34. Budarf ML, Konkle BA, Ludlow LB, Michaud D, Yamashiro DA, McDonald McGinn D, Zackai EH, Driscoll DA: Identification of a patient with a Bernard-Soulier syndrome and a deletion in the DiGeorge/Velo-cardio-facial chromosomal region in 22q11.2. Hum Mol Genet 1995; 4: 763-6.

35. Ludlow LB, Schick BP, Budarf ML, Driscoll DA, Zackai EH, Cohen A, Konkle BA: Identification of a mutation in a GATA binding site of the platelet glycoprotein Ibβ promoter resulting in the Bernard-Soulier syndrome. J Biol Chem 1996; 271: 22076-80.

36. Wright SD, Michaelides K, Johnson DJD, West NC, Tuddenham EGD: Double heterozygosity for mutations in the platelet glycoprotein IX gene in three siblings with Bernard-Soulier syndrome. Blood 1993; 81: 2339-47.

37. Clemetson J, Kyrie PA, Brenner B, Clemetson KJ: Variant Bernard-Soulier syndrome associated with a homozygous mutation in the leucine-rich domain of glycoprotein IX. Blood 1994; 84: 1124-31.

38. Ware J, Russell SR, Marchese P, Murata M, Mazzucato M, De Marco L, Ruggeri ZM: Point mutation in a leucine-rich repeat of platelet glycoprotein Ibα resulting in the Bernard-Soulier syndrome. J Clin Invest 1993; 92: 1213-20.

39. Miller JL, Lyle VA, Cunningham D: Mutation of leucine-57 to phenylalanine in a platelet glycoprotein Ibα leucine tandem repeat occurring in patients with an autosomal dominant variant of Bernard-Soulier disease. Blood 1992; 79: 439-46.

40. De La Salle C, Baas M-J, Lanza F, Schwartz A, Hanau D, Chevalier J, Gachet C, Briquel ME, Cazenave JP: A three-base deletion removing a leucine residue in a leucine-rich repeat of platelet glycoprotein Ibα associated with a variant of Bernard-Soulier syndrome (Nancy I). Br J Haematol 1995; 89: 386-96.

41. Kunishima S, Lopez JA, Kobayashi S, Imai N, Kamiya T, Saito H, Naoe T: Missense mutations of the glycoprotein (GP) Ibβ gene impairing the GPIb α/β disulfide linkage in a family with giant platelet disorder. Blood 1997; 89: 2404-12.

42. Humphries JE, Yirinec BA, Hess CE: Atherosclerosis and unstable angina in Bernard-Soulier syndrome. Am J Clin Pathol 1992; 97: 652-5.

43. Nieuwenhuis HK, Sakariassen KS, Houdijk WPM, Nievelstein PFEM, Sixma JJ: Deficiency of platelet membrane glycoprotein Ia associated with a decreased platelet adhesion to subendothelium: A defect in platelet spreading. Blood 1986; 68: 692-5.

44. Moroi M, Jung SM, Okuma M, Shinmyozu K: A patient with platelets deficient in glycoprotein VI that lack both collagen-induced aggregation and adhesion. J Clin Invest 1989; 84: 1440-5.

45. Polgar J, Clemetson JM, Kehrel BE, Wiedemann M, Magnenat EM, Wells TNC, Clemetson KJ: Platelet activation and signal transduction by convulxin, a C-type lectin from Crotalus durissus terrificus (tropical rattlesnake) venom via the p62/GPVI collagen receptor. J Biol Chem 1997; 272: 13576-83.

46. Kritzik M, Savage B, Nugent DJ, Santoso S, Ruggeri ZM, Kunicki TJ: Nucleotide polymorphisms in the α_2 gene define multiple alleles that are associated with differences in $\alpha_2\beta_1$ density. Blood 1998; 92: 2382-8.

47. Santoro SA: Platelet surface collagen receptor polymorphisms: Variable receptor expression and thrombotic/hemorrhagic risk. Blood 1999; 93: 3575-7.

48. Daniel JL, Dangelmaier C, Jin J, Ashby B, Smith BJ, Kunapuli SP: Molecular basis for ADP-induced platelet activation. I. Evidence for three distinct ADP receptors on human platelets. J Biol Chem 1998; 273: 2024-9.

49. Gachet C, Cattaneo M, Ohlmann P, Hechler B, Lecchi A, Chevalier J, Cassel D, Mannucci PM, Cazenave JP: Purinoceptors on blood platelets: Further pharmacological and clinical evidence to suggest the presence of two ADP receptors. Br J Haematol 1995; 91: 434-44.

50. Nurden P, Savi P, Heilmann E, Bihour C, Herbert JM, Maffrand JP, Nurden AT: An inherited bleeding disorder linked to a defective interaction between ADP and its receptor on platelets. J Clin Invest 1995; 95: 1612-22.

51. Levy-Toledano S, Maclouf J, Rosa JP, Gallet C, Valles G, Nurden P, Nurden AT: Abnormal tyrosine phosphorylation linked to a defective interaction between ADP and its receptor on platelets. Thromb Haemost 1998; 80: 463-8.

52. Hirata T, Ushikubi F, Kakizuka A, Okuma M, Narumiya S: Two thromboxane A2 receptor isoforms in human platelets. Opposite coupling to adenylate cyclase with different sensitivity to Arg^{60} to Leu mutation. J Clin Invest 1996; 97: 949-56.

53. Hayward CPM: Inherited disorders of platelet α-granules. Platelets 1997; 8: 197-209.

54. Weiss HJ, Lages B, Vicic W, Tsung LY, White JG: Heterogeneous abnormalities of platelet dense granule ultrastructure in 20 patients with congenital storage pool deficiency. Br J Haematol 1993; 83: 282-95.

55. Spritz RA: Molecular genetics of the Hermansky-Pudlak and Chediak-Higashi syndromes. Platelets 1998; 9: 21-9.

56. Dachary-Prigent J, Pasquet JM, Fressinaud E, Toti F, Freyssinet JM, Nurden AT: Aminophospholipid exposure, microvesiculation and abnormal protein tyrosine phosphorylation in the platelets of a patient with Scott syndrome: a study using physiologic agonists and local anaesthetics. Br J Haematol 1997; 99: 959-67.

3
FACTOR V: DR. JECKYLL AND MR. HYDE

Michael Kalafatis, Ph.D[1,2]
and Kenneth G. Mann, Ph.D[3]

From the [1]Department of Chemistry, Cleveland State University, Cleveland OH 44115, [2]Department of Molecular Cardiology, Lerner Research Institute, Cleveland Clinic Foundation, Cleveland OH 44195, email: m.kalafatis@csuohio.edu

[3]Department of Biochemistry, College of Medicine, University of Vermont, Burlington VT 05405 email; kmann@protein.med.uvm.edu

Key Words: Factor V, thrombosis, prothrombinase

Abstract:
The regulation of the delicate balance between the procoagulant and anticoagulant mechanisms is of extreme importance for survival. The procoagulant enzymatic complexes (i.e. prothrombinase, intrinsic tenase and extrinsic tenase) are similar in structure and composed of an enzyme, a cofactor, and the substrate associated on a cell surface in the presence of divalent metal ions. Factor Va and factor VIIIa, which are very similar in structure and function, are required for prothrombinase and intrinsic tenase activities respectively because both cofactors express a dual function in their respective complexes, acting as an enzyme receptor and catalytic effector on the cell surface. The cofactors derive from inactive plasma precursors by regulatory proteolytic events, which involve α-thrombin. In general bleeding tendencies are usually associated with defects in the activation of one of the zymogens or the cofactors of the procoagulant complexes. α-Thrombin, participates in its own down-regulation by binding to the endothelial cell receptor thrombomodulin, and initiating the protein C pathway, which in turn leads to the formation of activated protein C (APC). APC is required for efficient neutralization of factor Va cofactor activity which results in the inactivation of the prothrombin-activating complex. This inactivation can only occur in the presence of the appropriate membrane surface. APC down-regulates the prothrombinase complex by cleaving specific peptide bonds on the heavy chain of factor Va which results in the dissociation of the A2 domain of factor Va from the rest of the molecule. Irregularities in the mechanism of inactivation of factor Va by APC, are associated with thrombotic risk, presumably due to sustained prothrombin activation.

INTRODUCTION

Following vascular injury, the blood clotting process is initiated in order to stop blood from leaking outside the vasculature. Blood clotting involves many proteins, which act in concert to produce the procoagulant enzyme α-thrombin, which in turn is responsible for the generation of the fibrin plug. While generation of the fibrin plug is required for the arrest of excessive bleeding, unregulated clotting will result in the occlusion of the vessels and thrombosis. Thus, the regulation of the delicate balance between the procoagulant and anticoagulant mechanisms is of extreme importance for survival. The maintenance of hemostasis in human blood is a complex event, requiring the controlled interaction of protease, zymogens, cofactors and inhibitors on surfaces presented to the blood by the platelets, blood cells and vessel wall. Procoagulant events are regulated and are localized to damaged regions of vessels. The factors, which regulate thrombin generation, are manifold, and diseases of abnormal coagulation are often associated either with defects in the pathway leading to thrombin or in the processes, which regulate thrombin production. Deficient or unrestricted thrombin generation can lead to bleeding (hemorrhage) or vessel occlusion (thrombosis, infarction, etc.), respectively. Thus, an understanding of the origins of hemorrhagic and thrombotic disease must be rooted in an understanding of the factors regulating the thrombin response.

Theories of blood coagulation have recognized that initiation of thrombin generation and clotting of plasma in vitro arises from a pathway, that is characterized by a series of reactions initiated by presentation of procoagulant surfaces to circulating blood (1-3). Every reaction in the series involves the activation of an inactive plasma protease precursor (zymogens) via limited proteolysis to an activated plasma protease. Each newly activated protease activates other zymogens later in the sequence, producing a string of activation processes which culminate in thrombin generation and subsequent clot formation. Subsequent investigations described the architecture of each active enzyme at the procoagulant surface as an assembly, requiring calcium, of the active protease with a cofactor also activated by minor proteolysis. Common to each vitamin K-dependent zymogen relevant to coagulation is a highly-conserved NH_2-terminal "Gla-domain," which binds multiple calcium ions and contains 9-12 γ-carboxyglutamic acid residues. At the COOH-terminus is the serine protease domain, which is largely homologous to that of trypsin and chymotrypsin, with insertions which alter the macromolecular substrate specificity of each enzyme. Between the NH_2- and COOH-terminal domains is a region of the protein which varies in structure among the zymogens, containing either epidermal growth factor-like domains or kringle domains.

Tissue factor (TF) is now accepted as the in vivo initiator of thrombin generation in the revised theory of coagulation (4). The TF pathway proceeds by assembly of three distinct complexes. The first is the extrinsic tenase (factor VIIa and the membrane bound cofactor TF), which assembles when TF, normally sequestered from contact with the blood, encounters circulating factor VIIa because of an injury to the vasculature. The complex formed activates a fraction of the circulating zymogen factors X and IX to their respective active forms, factors Xa and IXa. The initial factor Xa produced potentiates cofactor activation, indirectly via limited thrombin generation. Factor IXa assembles with factor VIIIa to form the intrinsic tenase complex, which produces additional factor Xa. Free factor Xa assembles with factor Va into the prothrombinase complex on the cell surface, which is the activator of prothrombin to α-thrombin.

The enzymatic complex that activates prothrombin, termed prothrombinase, is composed of the serine protease factor Xa, and the cofactor, factor Va, associated on a cell membrane in the presence of Ca^{2+} (2,3). Historically factor V was identified as the activity in normal plasma that corrected the PT of plasma of a patient with factor V deficiency (5). Human factor V circulates in plasma at a concentration of 20 nM, as a large single chain procofactor with a M_r 330,000. Approximately 20% of the total human factor V found in whole human blood originate from the platelets α-granules (6). The significance of platelet factor V is underscored by either patients with a qualitative deficiency in platelet factor V (Factor V Quebec, 7) or by patients with circulating inhibitory factor V antibodies that have not access to platelet factor V (8).

Factor V is the precursor of factor Va which is the required cofactor of prothrombinase which in turn is responsible for the efficient catalysis of the activation of prothrombin to α-thrombin. Factor Va is required for prothrombinase activity because it serves a dual function, both as a factor Xa receptor and as a catalytic effector for factor Xa on a membrane or cell surface. Incorporation of factor Va into prothrombinase increases the rate at which prothrombin is converted to α-thrombin by 300,000-fold relative to the rate of the reaction produced by factor Xa alone (9).

As a consequence, irregularities in the mechanism of activation of factor V or a decrease in the concentration of factor V mostly results in bleeding disorders whereas abnormalities in the mechanism of inactivation of factor Va by APC are associated with thrombotic episodes because of sustained prothrombin activation. The physiological significance of factor Va for clot formation was demonstrated in mice where complete deficiency of factor V results in massive hemorrhage immediately after birth and consequent death (10). However, humans who are deficient in plasma factor V ($<$ 2% factor V clotting activity) have been described. Thus, platelet factor V is extremely important for normal hemostasis. The physiological relevance of factor Va in the generation of thrombosis is assured because of case reports of familial thrombophilia associated with factor V/Va mutations (11,12).

STRUCTURAL FEATURES AND REGULATION

The factor V gene is located on chromosome 1 at q21-25. The factor V gene is 80 kb in length, contains 24 introns and following transcription gives rise to a 6.8 kb mRNA (13). Synthesis of factor V has been demonstrated by bovine aortic endothelial cells, a human hepatocarcinoma cell line, HepG2, and by human and guinea pig megakaryocytes, the precursor cells of circulating platelets. The factor V antigen level in megakaryocytes has been shown to increase following treatment with PMA. This increase in antigen is at the protein level and is not associated with an increase in mRNA levels.

Factor V is cleaved by α-thrombin at Arg^{709}, Arg^{1018}, and Arg^{1545} to generate the active cofactor, and two heavily glycosylated activation peptides (14-16). The factor Va molecule is a heterodimer composed of a heavy chain of M_r 105,000 and a light chain of M_r 74,000. The two subunits are non-covalently associated via a divalent metal ion process. The cDNA and deduced amino acid sequence shows that the molecule contains triplicated "A" domains which share a high degree of homology with ceruloplasmin, duplicated "C" domains which share homology with discoidin and a connecting B region which functions as an activation peptide. The heavy chain contains the NH_2-terminus of the procofactor (residues 1-709) and is composed of two "A" domains (residues 1-303, and 317-656), connected by an amino acid region containing basic amino acids (residues 304-316). The COOH-terminal portion of the heavy chain (residues 657-709) is rich in acidic amino acids. The light chain of the cofactor contains the COOH-terminus of the factor V molecule (residues 1546-2196) and is composed of one "A" domain (residues 1546-1877) and two "C" domains (residues 1878-2036, and 2037-2196). Figure 1 depicts the structure of the three A domains based on the published coordinates of ceruloplasmin (17). The three conserved hydrophobic α loops are also identified. The highly hydrophobic nature of these loops and their conserved amino acid sequence are identified in figure 2. Figure 3 shows the ribbon structure of the A domains of factor V and the equivalent A domains in the homologous proteins, human factor VIII, and human ceruloplasmin.

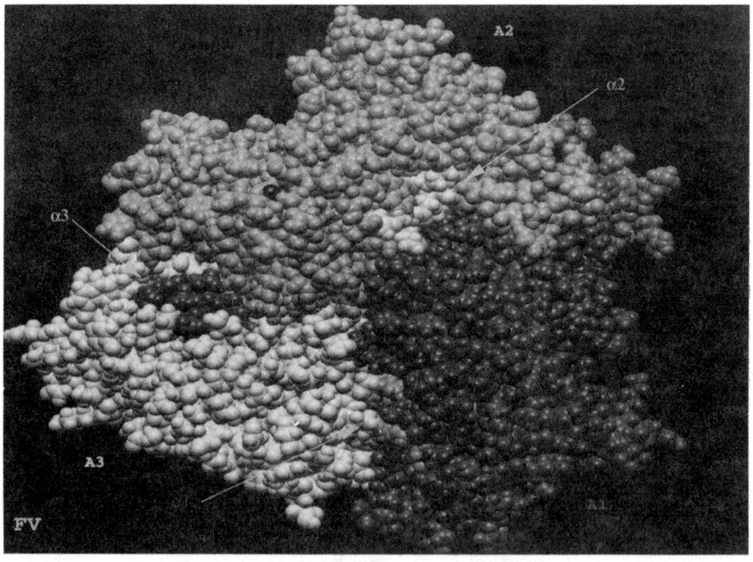

Figure 1. Structural analysis of the A domains of factor Va was performed by using as a template the known X-ray structure of ceruroplasmin (17). The position of the highly conserved α loops is also shown.

α1	FV:	139	CLTHIYYSHENLIEDFNSGLIGPLLIC	165
	FVIII:	153	CLTYSYLSHVDLVKDLNSGLIGALLVC	179
	Cp:	155	CVTRIYHSHIDAPKDIASGLIGPLIIC	181
α2	FV:	472	CLTRPYYSDVDIMRDIASGLIGLLLIC	498
	FVIII:	528	CLTRYYSSFVNMERDLASGLIGPLLIC	554
	Cp:	515	CLAKMYYSAVDPTKDIFTGLIGPMKIC	541
α3	FV:	1697	CRAWAYYSAVNPEKDIHSGLIGPLLIC	1723
	FVIII:	1832	CKAWAYFSDVDLEKDVHSGLIGPLLVC	1858
	Cp:	855	CIPWAYYSTVDQVKDLYSGLIGPLIVC	881

Figure 2. Amino acid sequence of the α loops in factor V, factor VIII, and ceruloplasmin.

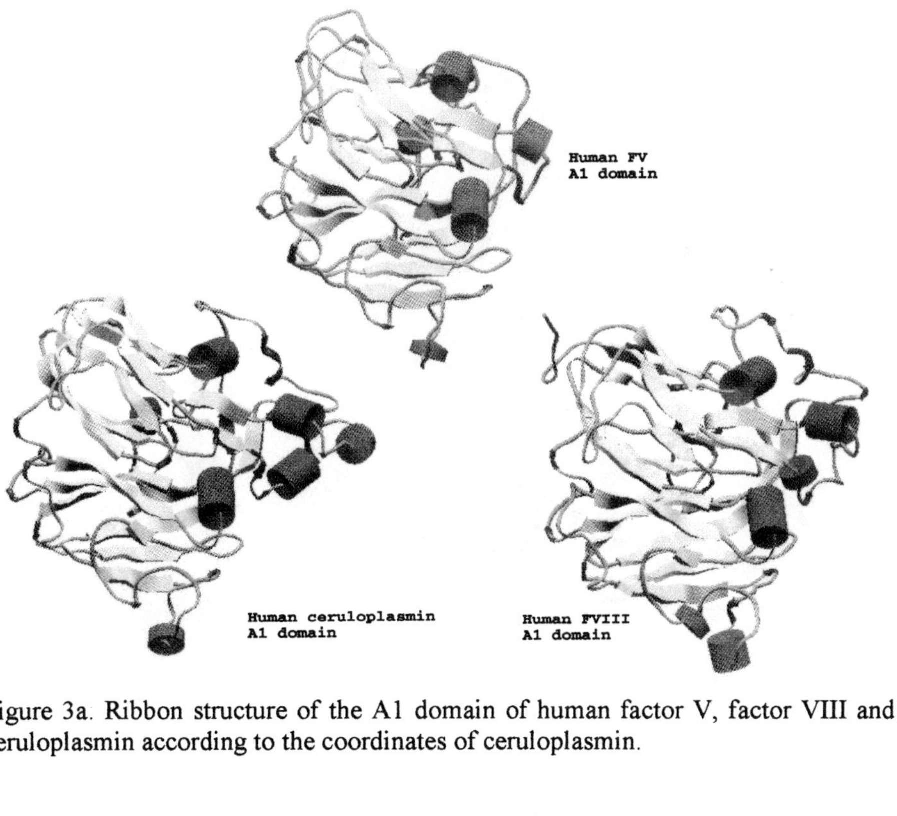

Figure 3a. Ribbon structure of the A1 domain of human factor V, factor VIII and ceruloplasmin according to the coordinates of ceruloplasmin.

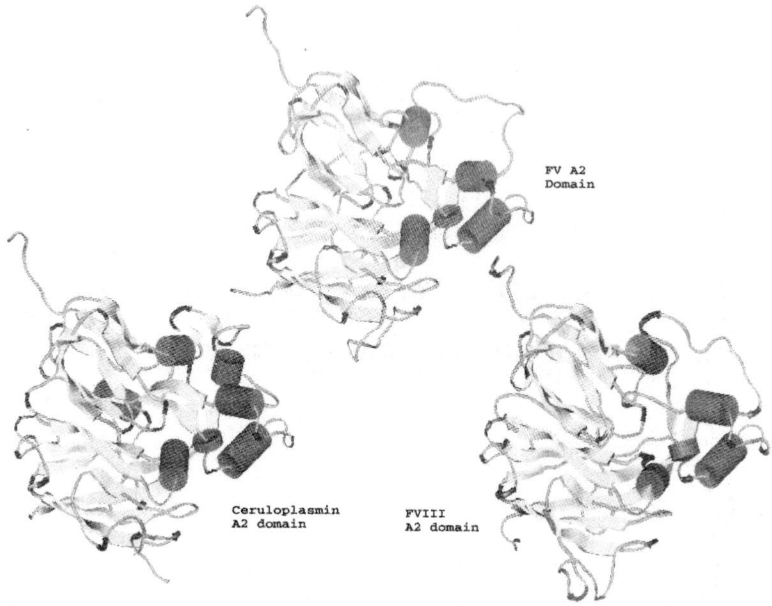

Figure 3b. Ribbon structure of the A2 domain of human factor V, factor VIII and ceruloplasmin according to the coordinates of ceruloplasmin.

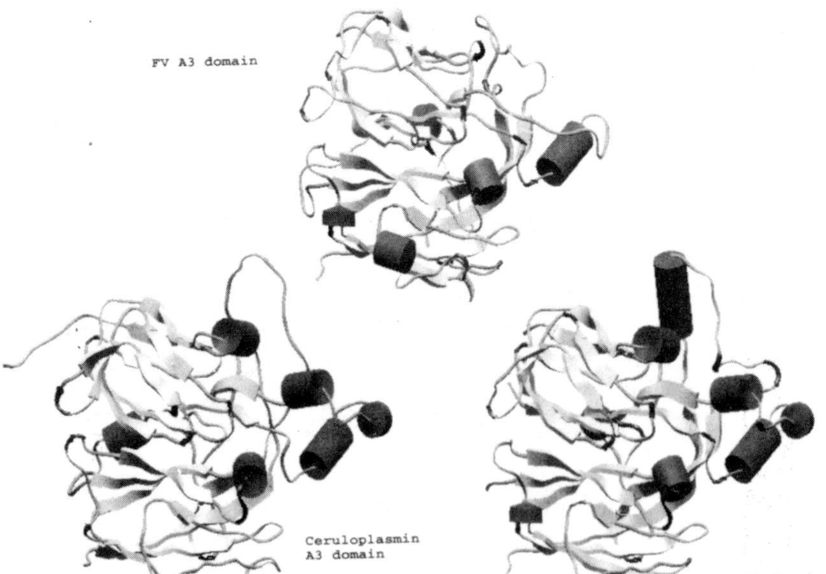

Figure 3c. Ribbon structure of the A3 domain of human factor V, factor VIII and ceruloplasmin according to the coordinates of ceruloplasmin.

Factor Va has 18 cysteine residues. Four of these cysteines are present as free -SH while the remaining fourteen are involved in disulfide bridges as follows (18,19): three 26 amino acid residue α-loops are present, one in each "A" domain; the "A1" and "A2" domains also contain one β-loop each of which composed of 82 amino acids; two γ-loops which are composed of 154 and 155 residues represent the "C1" and "C2" domains. The factor V molecule has multiple potential N-linked glycosylation sites in the B region and on the heavy and light chains that are required for secretion. The molecule is also phosphorylated by a membrane associated casein kinase II-like enzyme on the heavy chain (at Ser^{692}) and by a protein kinase C isoform on 2 sites of the light chain (20-22). Phosphorylation at Ser^{692} is required for fast and efficient inactivation of the cofactor by APC. Finally, Tyr^{665}, Tyr^{696},Tyr^{698}, Tyr^{1494}, Tyr^{1510}, Tyr^{1515}, and Tyr^{1565} are believed to be sulfated (23). Inhibition of sulfation by sodium chlorate results in a cofactor molecule 5-fold less active than the native molecule. It has been thus suggested that sulfation of factor V is important for α-thrombin activation of the procofactor. It has been also suggested that sulfation may by important for the interaction of factor Va with factor Xa.

α-Thrombin, the major procoagulant enzyme of the blood coagulation is also a major anticoagulant participating to its own down regulation. Once formed, α-thrombin binds to the endothelial cell receptor thrombomodulin and initiates the protein C pathway leading to the formation of activated protein C (APC). APC down-regulates α-thrombin generation by proteolytically inactivating factor Va and factor VIIIa and thus impairing their participation in the prothrombinase and tenase complexes respectively (24). However, under physiological conditions, inactivation of factor VIIIa occurs in the absence of APC following dissociation of the A2 domain of the cofactor (25,26). Hence APC is not essential for factor VIIIa inactivation. In contrast, proteolytic cleavage of factor Va by APC is required for complete inactivation of the cofactor and the arrest of its contribution to the procoagulant process (27,28). APC down-regulates the prothrombinase complex by cleaving specific peptide bonds on the heavy chain of factor Va which also results in the dissociation of the A2 domain of factor Va from the rest of the molecule. Dissociation of the A2 domain of both cofactors impairs their ability to interact with the other protein components of prothrombinase and intrinsic tenase and results in the arrest of α-thrombin formation. Interestingly, it has been demonstrated that effective down-regulation of α-thrombin generation by the protein C pathway in combination with TFPI and AT-III occurs because APC prevents the coexistence of the factor Va heavy and light chains (29).

The inactivation of human factor Va is membrane-dependent and occurs because of limited proteolysis by APC of the heavy chain at Arg^{506}, Arg^{306}, and Arg^{679} (27,28). The light chain of the cofactor is not cleaved by APC. The membrane dependent cleavage at Arg^{306} is required for complete inactivation. Phosphorylation of the cofactor by a platelet-membrane associated casein kinase II enzyme at the COOH-terminal portion of the heavy chain (at Ser^{692}) increases the rate of cofactor inactivation by APC because of acceleration of cleavage at Arg^{506}. It has been recently shown that upon cleavage at Arg^{306}/Arg^{506}, the A2 domain of the cofactor is dissociated from the rest of the molecule. The procofactor factor V is also inactivated by APC because of cleavages at Arg^{306}, Arg^{506}, Arg^{679}, and Lys^{994} (28). Cleavage at Arg^{306} in factor V is the inactivating cleavage site of the procofactor.

The bulk of data thus far accumulated clearly demonstrated that depending on the assay used and most precisely depending on the concentration of factor Xa used in each assay factor Va cleavages could sometimes be correlated with dramatic decrease in cofactor activity. A perfect example is illustrated by the inactivation of factor Va by APC (31). Cleavage at Arg^{306} is membrane dependent and responsible for the majority of the loss of factor Va activity independently of the assay used to measure cofactor activity (31). However, in the presence of saturating concentrations of factor Xa (>1 nM) in the absence of phospholipid vesicles, the human cofactor which is cleaved at Arg^{506} and Arg^{679} retains 60-80% of its cofactor activity. In contrast, when factor Va cofactor activity is assayed in a clotting assay (i.e. at 10 pM factor Xa) these cleavages result in the loss of the majority of the cofactor activity. It has been established that, APC cleaved-factor Va, in the absence of a membrane surface, has reduced affinity for factor Xa and prothrombin (30). These data demonstrate that the cleavages at Arg^{506} and Arg^{679} impair the cofactor's capability to interact with both factor Xa and prothrombin. The effective dissociation constant of membrane-bound factor Va cleaved at Arg^{506} and Arg^{679} (factor $Va_{506/679}$) for factor Xa is raised from 0.7 nM to 3.9 nM. As a consequence when measured at high factor Xa concentrations the cleavages at Arg^{506} and Arg^{679} (factor $Va_{506/679}$) reflect a moderate loss in the quantitative affinity for prothrombinase assembly rather than a total loss of factor Va cofactor activity. Upon addition of an anionic phospholipid surface, factor $Va_{506/679}$ is cleaved by APC at Arg^{306} to produce a cofactor molecule, factor $Va_{306/506/679}$, which is no longer capable of binding factor Xa. The latter loss of activity is concomitant with the dissociation of the A2 derived fragments from the rest of the molecule (31). The dissociation of the A2 domain from the rest of the factor Va molecule is thought to be the ultimate cause for the total loss of activity of the APC-cleaved factor Va molecules.

PHYSIOLOGICAL SIGNIFICANCE

Dahlbäck et al. (11) observed that plasma from an individual with venous thrombosis had an abnormal response to APC in a modified aPTT (activated Partial Thromboplastin Time) assay. When APC is introduced into normal plasma which has been preincubated with an aPTT reagent a prolongation of clotting time which is proportional to the concentration of APC used has been observed. In plasma from some patients, higher concentrations of APC are required to obtain similar prolongation of clotting time as seen with normal plasma. This condition was called "APC-resistance". The molecular defect in individuals with APC-resistance was identified at the genetic level by Bertina et al. (12) who showed that individuals with APC-resistance have a mutation in the factor V gene (a G to A substitution at nucleotide 1691). This mutation results in an $Arg^{506}\rightarrow Gln$ mutation in the factor V molecule. This mutation is present in up to 60% of patients with venous thrombosis and in 3-5% of normal individuals. As a consequence of the mutation the abnormal molecule, called factor V^{Leiden}, does not possess the APC-cleavage site at Arg^{506}

When isolated from the plasma of patients homozygous for the $Arg^{506}\rightarrow Gln$ mutation, factor Va^{Leiden} is inactivated by APC at a rate slower than that observed for normal factor Va (32). However, inactivation still proceeds as a consequence of cleavage at Arg^{306}. Interestingly, and in contrast to the observations made with factor Va^{Leiden}, the APC-catalyzed rate of inactivation of factor V^{Leiden} is comparable to that observed with normal factor V. These results are in agreement with the data demonstrating the initial membrane-dependent cleavage site in normal factor V which leads to inactivation occurs at Arg^{306}. The APC-catalyzed inactivation of membrane-bound factor V^{Leiden} also occurs through initial cleavage at Arg^{306} at a comparable rate to normal factor V, indicating that inactivation of factor V does not necessarily require cleavage at Arg^{506}. Recently, two independent groups reported patients with thrombotic disorders that were heterozygous for an amino acid substitution at the Arg^{306} cleavage site (33,34).

Dahlbäck et al. first reported that in patients with APC-resistance the defect could be overcome by the addition of normal plasma factor V and that the intact procofactor, single chain factor V, can act as a "cofactor" molecule contributing to the acceleration of inactivation of factor VIIIa by the APC/protein S complex (35). In contrast, factor V^{Leiden} was found to have a diminished "cofactor" effect for the inactivation of factor VIIIa by the APC/protein S complex (35). It was thus proposed that the thrombotic tendency in individuals with the $Arg^{506}\rightarrow Gln$ mutation may also be due to the loss of the "cofactor" activity of factor V which would result in delayed factor VIIIa inactivation and thus contribute to the increased thrombin generation observed in the plasma from APC-resistant individuals. We observed that factor V can accelerate the rate of factor VIII inactivation by APC, only in the presence of the intact form of protein S by approximately two-fold (26). APC-treated, membrane-bound factor V as well as α-thrombin activated factor Va (inclusive of the B domain) gave similar results. In contrast, purified factor Va (without the B domain) showed no cofactor effect on the rate of the inactivation of factor VIII by APC/protein S (36). These data suggest that a portion of the B region of the procofactor facilitates the inactivation of factor VIII only in the presence of the intact form of protein S. Recently we have confirmed this findings (37). Our data suggest that the B-domain fragments of factor V play a role for factor VIII inactivation and that APC and the B domain may interact at a 1:1 stoichiometry. Our data are in disagreement with recent reports suggesting that the cofactor effect of factor V is only observed when the B-domain of factor V is attached to the light chain of the cofactor (38). In contrast we found that the light chain alone is a inhibitor of the inactivation process of both factor Va and factor VIII by APC (39).

Usually the presence of a DNA mutation is frequently used to define a disease or a risk state. Since DNA typing has become easy and convenient in contrast to protein characterization, it is generally assumed that a mutation if present (or not) at the DNA level will be also present (or not) in the corresponding protein. However, discrepancies between the phenotype and the genotype can occur. Although the $Arg^{506}\rightarrow Gln$ substitution in the factor V molecule is by far the most common single point mutation which can be related to thrombosis, it remains puzzling that correlation of the mutation (at the genetic level) with a clear defined pathology (phenotypically) is yet to be established. Thus, since the presence of the mutation is not always associated with a disease state, it may be concluded that the abnormal allele may not always be equivalently expressed. The existence of other compensatory mutations in individuals with APC-resistance that could influence the APC sensitivity of factor V should not be excluded.

We have evaluated two individuals who are genetically heterozygous for the factor V^{Leiden} mutation. While these individuals, both symptomatic for thrombotic episodes, are genetically heterozygous for factor V^{Leiden} they are phenotypically homozygous, displaying only the factor V^{Leiden} allele. The form of factor V expressed in the patients' blood was evaluated following clotting and APC/PCPS cleavage. Our data demonstrate absence of correlation between the genotype at position 1691 and the corresponding phenotype data in patients with pseudohomozygous factor V^{Leiden}, suggesting the existence of heterogeneous genetic lesions which interfere with factor V expression, processing secretion and/or stability. Since the presence of the factor V^{Leiden} molecule in plasma is directly related to the pathology, visualization of the form of factor V in whole plasma is required for the diagnosis of individuals with APC-resistance (40).

Since factor Va^{Leiden} is inactivated by APC with a rate slower than normal factor Va, patients who posses both factor Va^{Leiden} and a mutation in the factor VIII molecule, which would classify them as hemophiliacs, may have a milder bleeding syndrome than hemophiliac patients with normal factor V and a similar defect in the factor VIII molecule. Nichols et al. reported significant differences in pathology among two sets of unrelated patients carrying the same factor VIII missense mutations (41). These mutations usually result in a phenotype characterized as severe hemophilia A. However, while two patients carrying the normal factor V gene were classified clinically as severe hemophiliacs, two others heterozygous for the $Arg^{506} \rightarrow Gln$ mutation, were classified as mild/moderate hemophiliacs. These results were based on the level of measurable FVIII activity in a one-stage clotting assay using factor VIII deficient plasma. The effect of a factor VIII deficiency is a reduced α-thrombin formation rate, whereas in the case of factor V^{Leiden}, the effect is an increase in α-thrombin formation. It appears that in the case of these two combined deficiencies, the extended lifetime of the abnormal factor Va molecule (factor Va^{Leiden}) is able to partially compensate for the abnormal factor VIII molecule resulting in sufficient α-thrombin generation to provide hemostasis. However, in humans there are reports of individuals with very low levels of factor V antigen and activity that have mild bleeding symptoms. Increased α-thrombin generation in a hemophiliac population that are heterozygous for factor V^{Leiden} was recently demonstrated in vitro (42).

Following injury to the vasculature the temporary structural integrity of the vessel is ensured by the fibrin clot which is composed of insoluble fibrin polymers and activated platelets. Removal of the fibrin clot is accomplished by the fibrinolytic cascade which results in plasminogen activation. We have shown that for a given concentration of APC, clot lysis is considerably delayed in plasma from individuals homozygous for the $Arg^{506} \rightarrow Gln$ substitution when compared to clot lysis in normal plasma (43). These data suggest that resistance of factor Va^{Leiden} to inactivation by APC may also result in sustained α-thrombin formation which in turn will enhance activation of TAFI. As a consequence removal of the fibrin clot would be impaired.

Thus, individuals with factor V^{Leiden} not only will have a tendency to clot more than individuals with normal factor V because of continuous activation of prothrombin, but also once formed the clot will be more resistant to fibrinolysis because of sustained activation of TAFI. Our findings were confirmed by Broze and Higushi who demonstrated premature lysis of clots from hemophilic plasma (44).

REFERENCES

1. Morawitz P. Die Chemie der Blutgerrnnum. Ergenbn Physiol. 1905;4:307-423.

2. Kalafatis M, Egan JO, van't Veer C, Cawthern M, and Mann KG. The regulation of clotting factors. Critical Reviews in Eukariotic Gene Expression 1997;**7**, 241-280.

3. Mann KG, Nesheim ME, Church WR, Haley P, and Krishnaswamy S. Surface-dependent reactions of the vitamin K-dependent enzyme complexes. Blood, 1990; 76, 1-16.

4. Gailani D, Broze GJ Jr: Factor XI activation in a revised model of blood coagulation. Science 1991;253, 909-912.

5. Owren PA. Parahemophilia: haemorragic diathesis due to absence of a previously unknown clotting factor. Lancet 1947; 1993: 446-448.

6. Tracy PB, Eide LL, Bowie EJW, Mann KG. Radioimmunoassay of factor V in human plasma and platelets. Blood 1982;60, 59-63.

7. Tracy PB, Giles AR, Mann KG, Eide LL, Hoogendoorn H, and Rivard GE. Factor V (Quebec): a bleeding diathesis associated with a qualitative platelet factor V deficiency. J. Clin. Invest. 1984;74, 1221-1228.

8. Nesheim ME, Nichols WL, Cole TL, Houston JG, Schenk RB, Mann KG, and Bowie EJW. Isolation and Study of an acquired inhibitor of human coagulation factor V. J. Clin. Invest. 1986;77, 405-415.

9. Nesheim ME, Taswell JB, Mann KG. The contribution of bovine factor V and factor Va to the activity of prothrombinase. J Biol Chem 1979; 254: 10952-10962.

10. Cui J O'Shea KS, Purkayastha A, Sauders TL, Ginsburg D. Fatal haemorrhage and incomplete block to embryogenesis in mice lacking coagulation factor V. Nature 1996;384, 66-68.

11. Dahlbäck B, Carlsson M, Svensson PJ. Familial thrombophilia due to a previously unrecognized mechanism characterized by poor anticoagulant response to activated protein C. Prediction of a cofactor to activated protein C. Proc. Natl. Acad. Sci. USA 1993;90, 1004-1008.

12. Bertina RM, Koeleman BPC, Koster T, Rosendaal FR, Dirven RJ, de Ronde H, van der Velden PA, Reitsma PH. Mutation in blood coagulation factor V associated with resistance to activated protein C. Nature 1994; 369: 64-67.

13. Cripe LD, Moore KD, Kane WH. Structure of the gene for human coagulation factor V. *Biochemistry* 1992; 31: 3777-3785.

14. Nesheim ME, and Mann KG (1979): Thrombin-catalyzed activation of single factor V. *J. Biol. Chem.* 254, 1326-1334.

15. Esmon CT (1979): The subunit structure of thrombin-activated factor V. Isolation of activated factor V, separation of subunits and reconstitution of biological activity. *J. Biol. Chem.* 254, 964-973.

16. Suzuki K, Dahlback B, Stenflo J (1982): Thrombin-catalyzed activation of human coagulation factor V. J. Biol. Chem. 257, 6556-6564.

17. Villoutreix BO, and Dahlback B. Stuctural investigation of the A domains of human blood coagulation factor V by molecular modeling. Protein Science 1998;7, 1317-1325.

18. Xue J, Kalafatis M, Mann KG. Determination of the disulfide bridges in factor Va light chain. Biochemistry 1993; 32: 5917-5923.

19. Xue J, Kalafatis M, Silveira JR, Kung C, Mann KG. Determination of the disulfide bridges in factor Va heavy chain. Biochemistry 1994; 33: 13109-13116.

20. Kalafatis M, Rand MD, Jenny RJ, Ehrlich YH, Mann KG. Phosphorylation of factor Va and factor VIIIa by activated platelets. Blood 1993; 81: 704-719.

21. Rand MD, Kalafatis M, Mann KG. Platelet coagulation factor Va: The major secretory platelet phosphoprotein. Blood 1994; 83: 2180-2190.

22. Kalafatis M. Identification and partial characterization of factor Va heavy chain kinase from human platelets. J. Biol. Chem. 1998; 273, 8459-8466.

23. Hortin GL. Sulfation of tyrosine residues in coagulation factor V. Blood 1993; 76: 946-952.

24. Esmon CT (1987): The regulation of natural anticoagulant pathways. Science 235 1348-1352.

25. Lollar P, Parker CG. pH-dependent denaturation of thrombin-activated porcine factor VIII. J. Biol. Chem. 1990; 265, 1688-1692.

26. Lu D, Kalafatis M, Mann KG, Long GL (1996): Comparison of activated protein S-mediated inactivation of human factor VIII and factor V. Blood 87, 4708-4717.

27. Kalafatis M, Mann KG. Role of the membrane in the inactivation of factor Va by activated protein C. J Biol Chem 1993; 268: 27246-27257.

28. Kalafatis M, Rand, MD, Mann KG. The mechanism of inactivation of human factor V and human factor Va by activated protein C. J Biol Chem; 1994; 269: 31869-31880.

29. van't Veer Cornelis, Golde NJ, Kalafatis M, and Mann KG. Inhibitory Mechanism of the protein C pathway on tissue factor-induced thrombin generation. Synergistic effect in combination with tissue factor pathway inhibitor. J. Biol. Chem 1997; 272, 7983-7994.

30. Mann KG, Hockin MF, Begin KJ, Kalafatis M. Activated protein C cleavage of factor Va leads to dissociation of the A2 domain. J. Biol. Chem. 1997; 272, 20678-20683.

31. Hockin MF, Kalafatis M, Shatos M, Mann KG. Protein C activation and factor V inactivation on human umbilical vein endothelial cells. Arterioscler. Thromb. Vasc. Biol. 1997; 17: 2765-2775.

32. Kalafatis M, Bertina RM, Rand MD, Mann KG. Characterization of the molecular defect in factor V^{R506Q}. J Biol Chem 1995; 270: 4053-4057.

33. Williamson D, Brown K, Luddington R, Baglin C, Baglin T (1998): Factor V Cambridge: A

new mutation (Arg^{306}-Thr) associated with resistance to activated protein C. Blood 1998;91: 1140-1144.

34. Chan WP, Lee CK, Kwong YL, Lam CK, Liang R (1998): A novel mutation of Arg^{306} of factor V gene in Hong Kong Chinese. Blood 1998;91: 1135-1139.

35. Shen L, Dahlbäck B. Factor V and protein S as synergistic cofactors to activated protein C in degradation of factor VIIIa. J Biol Chem 1994; 269: 18735-18738.

36. Varadi K, Rosing J, Tans I, Pabinger I, Keil B, Schwarz HP. Factor V enhances the cofactor function of protein S in the APC-mediated inactivation of factor VIII: Influence of the factor V^{R506Q} mutation. Thromb. Haemost 1996; 76: 208-214.

37. Kalafatis M and Mann KG. Contributions of the B region of factor V to the inactivation of factor VIII by Activated Protein C (APC). Thromb. Haemost 1999; 82: 742a.

38. Thorelli E, Kaufman RJ, Dahlback B. Cleavage of factor V at Arg506 by activated protein C and the expression of anticoagulant activity of factor V. Blood 1999; 93: 2552-2558.

39. Hockin MF, Cawthern KM, Kalafatis M, and Mann KG. A model describing the inactivation of factor Va by APC: bond cleavage, fragment dissociation, and product inhibition. Biochemistry 1999; 38: 6918-6934.

40. Kalafatis M, Bernardi F, Simioni P, Lunghi B, Girolami A, and Mann KG. Phenotype and Genotype Expression in Pseudohomozygous factor V^{Leiden}. The need for phenotype analysis. Arterioscler. Thromb. Vasc. Biol. 1999; 19: 336-342.

41. Nichols WC, Amano K, Cacheris PM, Figueiredo MS, Michaelides K, Schwaab R, Hoyer L, Kaufman RJ, Ginsburg D. Moderation of hemophilia A phenotype by the factor V R506Q mutation. Blood 1996; 88: 1183-1187.

42. vant'Veer C, Golden NJ, Simioni P, Bertina RM, and Mann KG. An in vitro analysis of the combination of Hemophilia A and factor V^{Leiden}. Blood 1997; 90: 3067-3072.

43. Bajzar L, Kalafatis M, Simioni P, Tracy PB. An antifibrinolytic mechanism describing the prothrombotic effect associated with factor V^{LEIDEN}. J Biol Chem 1996; 271: 22949-22952.

44. Broze GJ Jr, Higuchi DA (1996): Coagulation-dependent inhibition of fibrinolysis: role of carboxypeptidase-U and the premature lysis of clots from hemophilic plasma. Blood; 1996:88, 3815-3823.

4

GENE THERAPY FOR HEMOPHILIA B: AAV-MEDIATED TRANSFER OF THE GENE FOR COAGULATION FACTOR IX TO HUMAN MUSCLE

Peter J. Larson, M.D., and Katherine A. High, M.D.

Department of Pediatrics, University of Pennsylvania School of Medicine, The Children's Hospital of Philadelphia, PA 19104

Hemophilia B is an X-linked bleeding disorder caused by a deficiency of coagulation factor IX. In its severe form, the disease results in spontaneous bleeding as well as bleeding following surgery or trauma, and is clinically indistinguishable from hemophilia A (factor VIII deficiency). The major morbidity of the disease is the chronic arthropathy of hemophilia that develops following spontaneous hemorrhage into the joint spaces. Blood in the joint space serves as an irritant causing proliferation of the vascular synovial membranes. Hypertrophied synovium is more susceptible to injury resulting in a vicious cycle of rebleeding that furthers the destruction of the joint. The major bleeding-related mortality of hemophilia is intracranial hemorrhage that occurs in between 3 and 14% of patients (1-3). The mortality rate from intracranial hemorrhage ranges from 20-50%, and survivors are often left with severe neurological sequelae such as seizures, paresis or mental retardation (1). Current treatment of hemophilia is based on the episodic intravenous infusion of highly purified plasma-derived or recombinant clotting factor concentrates in response to bleeding episodes (on-demand therapy).

A gene transfer approach to the treatment of hemophilia has been long awaited as a means to obviate the need for chronic infusion therapy. Two important observations derived from over 40 years of experience with clotting factor replacement therapy provide the rationale for a gene therapy approach to the treatment of hemophilia. The first is based on the experience of patients treated on primary prophylaxis regimens. With such regimens, patients are begun on regular infusions of coagulation factor at an early age with a goal of maintaining trough levels of factor VIII or factor IX of at least 1% (4, 5). This approach, pioneered by Swedish hemophilia treaters, preserves joint radiographic status and function, and minimizes serious bleeding complications. If transfer of a functional factor IX gene is successful in raising the blood levels of factor IX to only 1% of normal, it is

Hemophilia Care in the New Millennium, edited by D. Monroe *et al.*
Kluwer Academic/Plenum Publishers, 2001

anticipated that patients may enjoy the same therapeutic benefits that attend prophylaxis regimens. The second compelling reason for gene transfer for hemophilia relates to the limitations associated with the factor concentrates themselves. Factor concentrates are expensive. The cost of treating an adult with severe hemophilia on demand is between $50,000-$300,000 per year. Infusion therapy is also inconvenient in that it requires gaining intravenous access. More importantly, in the 1960s, 1970s, and 1980s the contamination of the blood supply, from which factor concentrates were produced, resulted in the infection of many patients with the hepatitis B and C and HIV viruses. Although products derived from plasma that are used today are safe with respect to lipid enveloped viruses, product recalls have occurred recently due to the concern about other potentially infectious agents such as prions that result in transmissible spongiform encephalopathy, and non-lipid encapsulated viruses such as hepatitis A and parvo B19 viruses (6-8). In addition, previously unknown agents that contaminate the blood supply continue to be described (9-11). A gene therapy approach should eliminate the risk of inadvertent transmission of these agents due to therapy.

Hemophilia is a good model for gene therapy for several reasons. First, precise regulation of expression of the donated gene is not required. The data from primary prophylaxis studies imply that levels as low as 1-2% may be beneficial in preventing complications of the disease. In addition, experience with the use of highly purified coagulation factor concentrates suggests that if gene transfer were so efficient as to result in plasma levels of factor of over 100%, such levels would not result in thrombosis. This is partly explained by the fact that these proteins circulate in an inactive form, and that activation and activity of the coagulation system are highly regulated events occurring at or near the site of vascular injury. Thus, the therapeutic window is wide, ranging from 1-100%. Second, tissue specific expression is not required. As long as the coagulation protein expressed in a particular tissue undergoes the critical post-translational processing events that lead to activity and can gain access to the circulation, any tissue type would be a potential target for gene transfer. Third, two well characterized animal models exist for hemophilia, naturally occurring dog models (12, 13) and the engineered factor VIII and factor IX knock-out mice (14, 15). Finally, determination of therapeutic effect is straightforward since the aPTT and factor IX activity levels can be readily measured in most laboratories.

Adeno-associated viral (AAV) vectors have been developed from the type 2 adeno-associated virus, a non-enveloped replication-defective parvovirus (16). To make AAV vector, all viral coding sequence (~4.7 kb) between the two flanking inverted terminal repeats is deleted and replaced with regulatory sequences and the transgene of interest (figure 1). AAV has the advantage that it does not require dividing target cells to achieve efficient transduction (17-19). In addition, because all of the viral genes have been removed, there is no immune response against the transduced cells due to the expression of viral proteins. These characteristics explain, in part, the long term (~2 years) expression *in vivo* from AAV transduced cells following a single administration of the vector [(19), and unpublished data]. The vector has several limitations. First, it cannot accommodate inserts larger that ~4.5 kb thus limiting its use for factor VIII deficiency where the cDNA is ~7 kb, or ~4.5 kb for B-domain deleted factor VIII. In addition, for a number of years, AAV vector was difficult to produce in large quantities, limiting accumulation of *in vivo* efficacy data.

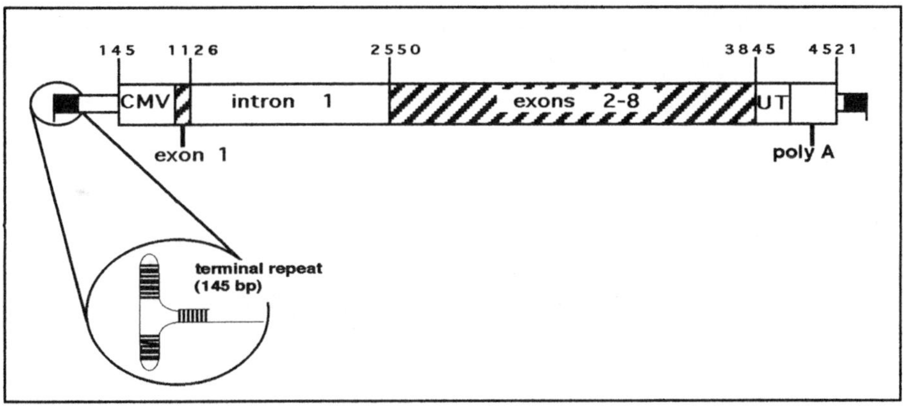

Fig. 1. Diagram of AAV-hFIX.

Skeletal muscle offers several advantages over other tissues as a target for gene therapy for hemophilia. Since fibers in most muscle groups survive for the lifetime of the organism, stable transduction of muscle has the potential to result in prolonged if not lifelong expression of factor IX (20). Skeletal muscle is a well-vascularized tissue affording ready access of secreted proteins into the circulation, and in humans a substantial muscle mass is available for transduction. A particular benefit of muscle as a target tissue for gene therapy for hemophilia is the ease of vector administration, which can be accomplished by percutaneous injection obviating the need for surgery and its attendant risks of bleeding complications. In addition, most patients with severe hemophilia over the age of 15 are infected with hepatitis B or C viruses. Many investigators feel that this makes liver a less desirable target tissue because of the theoretical risks related to increased carcinogenesis (effect of pre-existing hepatitis, combined with therapy with an integrating vector), and increased risk of inhibitor formation in the milieu of altered cytokine production with chronic hepatitis.

In pre-clinical studies, our group has demonstrated that therapeutic levels (5-7%) of factor IX can be expressed in mice following a single administration of AAV vector. In these experiments, hindlimb muscles of C57Bl/6 and Rag-1 mice were injected with AAV vector encoding human factor IX. In the immunocompetent (C57Bl/6) mice, immunofluorescence staining of muscle harvested 3 months after injection demonstrated the presence of human factor IX intracellularly and in the surrounding extracellular matrix. No human factor IX was detected in the C57Bl/6 plasma due to the formation of antibodies to human factor IX. Results of similar experiments in immunodeficient (Rag-1) mice demonstrated therapeutic levels of human factor IX in the plasma (~250-350 ng/mL or 5-7%) (figure 2). In the Rag-1 mice, factor IX expression increased over a period of weeks before reaching a plateau that was stable for up to 67 weeks following injection. In addition, as is evident in the figure, the expression was dose-dependent.

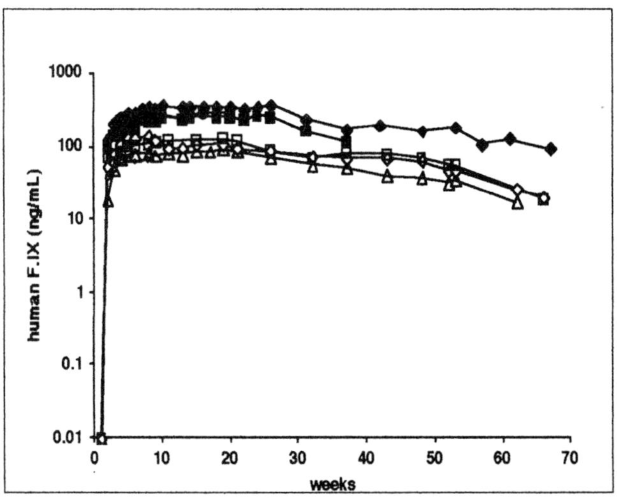

Fig. 2. Plasma levels in Rag-1 mice after intramuscular injection of AAV-hFIX. Levels from mice injected IM with 10^{13} vector genomes (v.g.)/kg are shown in the upper series of lines, and with 5×10^{11} v.g./kg in the lower series. Each line represents levels from a single animal.

Prior to initiating a trial of gene transfer in humans, important issues relating to therapy should be addressed first in a large animal model of the disease. Dogs with factor IX deficiency caused by a point mutation in the portion of the gene encoding the heavy chain of the factor IX molecule are maintained in the dog colony in Chapel Hill, NC. These dogs have severe factor IX deficiency (levels <1%), and have a clinical phenotype that mirrors the human disease. Unlike the inbred strains of mice used in preliminary experiments, the canine model of hemophilia has allowed for the characterization of the immune response to the transgene product in an animal model that, like the human population, has a more heterogenous immune system. In addition, it is necessary to refine vector production in order to produce adequate amounts to treat humans. Scale up of recombinant vector production from the mouse (20 gr) to the dog (20-40 kg) represents a 400-800 fold increase. Accomplishing this, the scale up from dog to human will require only a 3-10 fold increase in production.

Table I. Dose response in hemophilia B dogs injected IM with AAV-cFIX vector

dog	**age**	**sex**	**vector dose/kg**	**# of sites**	**vol/ site**	**ave WBCT* [min]**	**ave aPTT* [sec]**	**ave plasma cFIX* [ng/ml]**
1	2 mo	M	$1.3x10^{11}$	18	250 μl	20.0	61.5	2.6
2	4 mo	M	$1.1x10^{12}$	8	375 μl	20.0	49.0	12.0
3	8 mo	F	$3.4x10^{12}$	60	300 μl	16.0	40.0	17.0
4	2 mo	F	$8.5x10^{12}$	24	500 μl	17.0	38.0	69.0
5	7 mo	M	$3.0x10^{12}$	28	500 μl	15.0	40.0	25.0

*Whole blood clotting times (WBCT) and activated thromboplastin times (aPTT) were >60 min and >50 sec, respectively, pre-injection for all five dogs. Average values after vector administration are determined after stabilization of factor IX levels. Values obtained during plasma infusion therapy are omitted. Normal aPTT=13.5-18 sec; normal WBCT=6-8 min.

Five dogs have been injected with increasing doses of recombinant AAV containing the transgene for canine factor IX. The study is ongoing, and between 40 weeks and 24 months of follow-up data are currently available for analysis. All dogs underwent multiple injections on a single occasion into muscles in the hindlimb. In some cases, injections were guided by ultrasound in order to minimize or prevent intravascular injection and inadvertent hematogenous dissemination of vector to non-target tissues. Injections were performed without prior replacement with canine factor IX (plasma), and only one dog had bleeding related to the injections. Local or systemic toxicity due to vector administration has not been observed. Efficacy has been assessed by measuring the levels of factor IX antigen in plasma, the aPTT, and by the whole blood clotting time (WBCT), an activity measure of low levels of factor IX that is more sensitive than the aPTT (Table I). Partial correction of the WBCT was observed in all dogs, and of the aPTT in four of the five dogs. Factor IX levels at plateau were dose dependent, ranging from 3 to 70 ng/mL (up to 1-2%). Levels of expression have not waned following the initial injections.

One of the five dogs developed an inhibitory antibody to canine factor IX. This inhibitor was low titer (<7 BU) and developed 2 weeks following vector administration. The inhibitor was transient and disappeared within two months, concurrent with a rise in factor IX levels in plasma and a shortening of the WBCT (figure 3). A second dog developed a transient non-inhibitory antibody at day 14 following injection that prolonged the WBCT for two weeks presumably due to more rapid clearance of circulating factor IX. These antibodies have not re-appeared in either dog.

An interpretation of these data requires the appreciation that treated animals were naïve with respect to exposure to factor IX; the dogs in the Chapel Hill colony have no circulating factor IX protein, and most animals had never been infused with canine plasma. In this regard they are similar to previously untreated patients (PUPs) treated with recombinant clotting factor concentrates. Transient inhibitors were first widely recognized in the PUP trials with recombinant factor VIII (rFVIII) because the study design included routine measurement of inhibitor titers. In these large PUP trials, the incidence of inhibitor formation was ~20% (21, 22), and for about half of these patients, the inhibitor was transient and decreased substantially or disappeared. Contemporary studies of the immune response to plasma-derived concentrates documented a similar phenomenon (23-25). Since inhibitors are usually sought only if the patient fails to respond to factor infusions, it is likely that such transient inhibitors were not detected before these studies. In preliminary data from trials of PUPs receiving recombinant factor IX concentrates, only 2 of 64 patients has developed a high-titer inhibitor (pers. comm. Suzanne Courter, Genetics Institute). Thus it appears that an antibody response is not uncommon on exposure to clotting factor, and in many cases is self-limited. In addition, the presence of infection or massive tissue injury at the time of exposure to clotting factor has been proposed as a factor in inhibitor development (26). Interestingly, the single dog that developed the inhibitory antibody was noted to have a skin infection at the time of injection with vector.

Given the remarkable safety profile in pre-clinical studies of AAV vector administered intramuscularly in animals, and the achievement of therapeutically

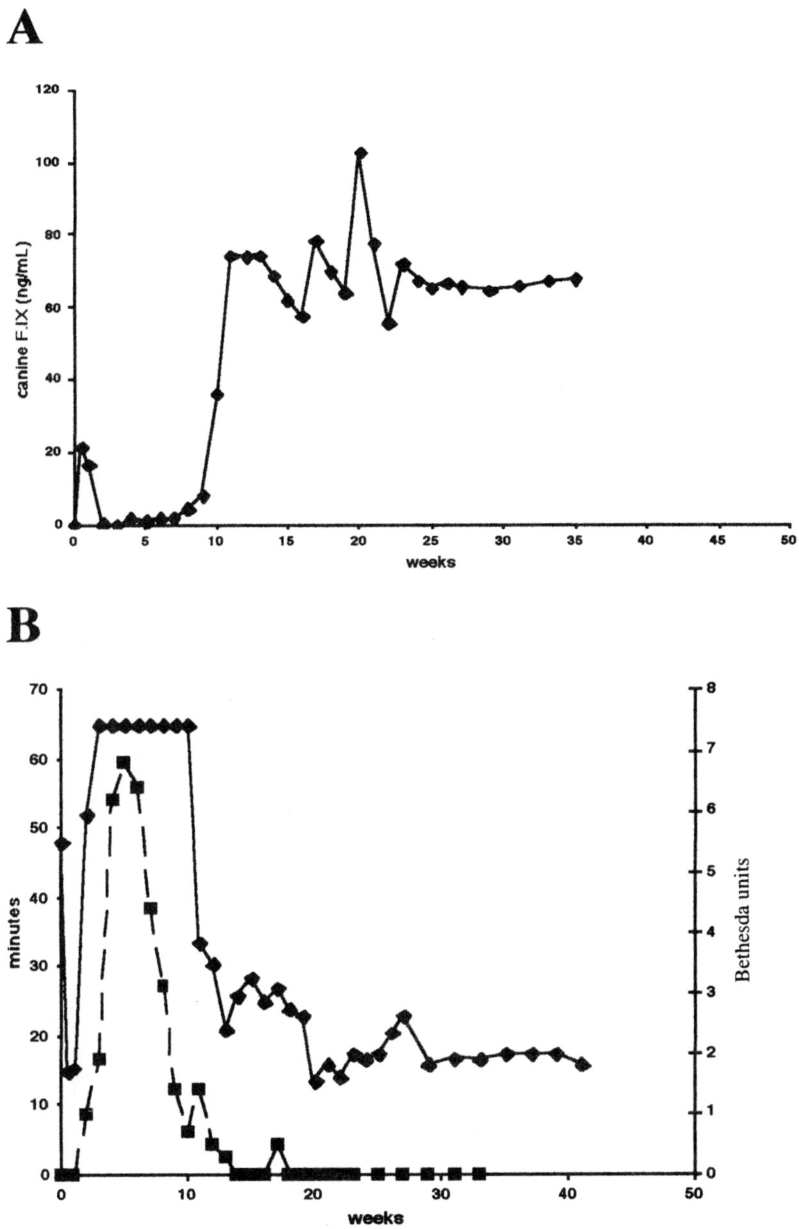

Fig. 3. Course of inhibitory antibody in a dog with hemophilia B following gene transfer. Panel A: Factor IX levels by ELISA. Panel B: dashed line plots the titer of the inhibitory antibody; solid line plots the whole blood clotting time.

meaningful levels of factor IX in animals injected with higher doses of vector, we have moved forward with a study of AAV containing the human factor IX transgene in patients with severe hemophilia B. This trial has been approved by review boards at the participating institutions, by the FDA under an Investigational New Drug Application, and by the Recombinant DNA Committee of the National Institutes of Health.

Table II. Dose groups in the phase I/II study

Group	**Patients**	**Injection Sites**	**Dose/kg (vector genomes)**
1	3	6-50	2.0×10^{11}
2	3	6-50	2.0×10^{12}
3	3	6-50	1.0×10^{13}

In this phase I/II dose escalation trial, we will enroll a total of at least 9 patients into 3 cohorts at increasing doses (Table II). Although the study is designed primarily to assess safety of the vector in humans, extrapolation of results observed in animals suggests that patients in groups 2 and 3 may achieve factor IX levels in the circulation of >1%. Such levels may be expected to improve the clinical phenotype of a patient with severe hemophilia. In addition, because the immune response following injection is unknown in humans but may preclude re-administration of vector, we have attempted to minimize the number of patients who will receive sub-therapeutic doses.

Eligible subjects will be admitted to the inpatient Clinical Research Center on the day of vector administration. Eligibility and exclusion criteria are detailed in Table III. Subjects will receive an initial dose of factor IX calculated to raise plasma levels to 100% of normal prior to injection and a 50% correction within the next 12 hours. Patients will remain hospitalized for 24 hours (or longer for bleeding or other unforeseen complications). During the hospitalization and for the balance of the study, patients will receive factor IX concentrate and other medications as clinically indicated. Injection of AAV-hFIX will be carried out with topical anesthesia or conscious sedation if necessary. All injections will be made into the *vastus lateralis* head of the *quadriceps* muscle (figure 4), so that vector is confined to a single well-circumscribed site in a muscle bundle that is not critical for *quadriceps* function or for stability of the knee joint. The *vastus lateralis* will be localized by ultrasound and injected at discrete intervals. During the procedure, the skin above 3 of the injection sites will be marked with a tattoo in order to facilitate localization of injection sites for subsequent muscle biopsies.

Detailed post-treatment evaluation will be carried out on each patient. The injection sites will be examined at each visit. Muscle biopsies will be obtained at 2, 6 and possibly 12 months, and tissue will be examined histologically for evidence of inflammation. Toxicity to organ systems (hepatic, renal, bone marrow, muscle) will be assessed by periodic physical examination and blood studies including complete

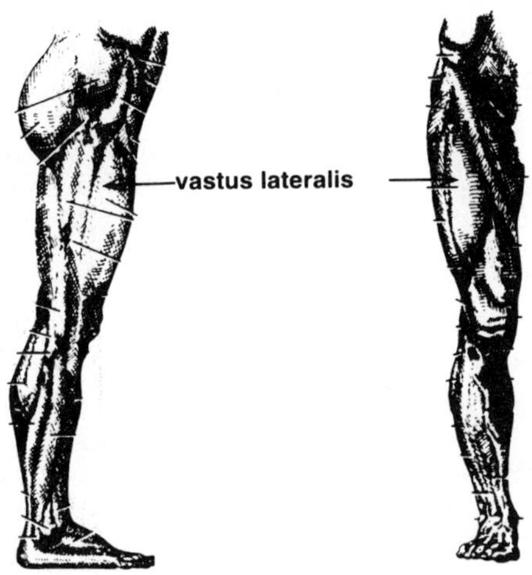

Fig. 4. Anatomy of the human lower extremity showing the *vastus lateralis* head of the *quadriceps* muscle.

blood counts, liver and renal function tests, urinalysis, and a muscle-specific marker, creatine phosphokinase. Efficiency of transfer of the factor IX gene into human muscle will be determined by isolating DNA from biopsied muscle and probing for vector sequences in order to estimate gene copy number. Expression of human factor IX in injected muscle tissue will be assessed using immunofluorescence staining. Factor IX activity and aPTTs will be measured by standard clinical assays. Human factor IX antigen levels will be determined by ELISA. In patients who have circulating baseline non-functional factor IX (CRM+), the whole blood clotting time (modified Lee-White time) will be followed until the aPTT shortens. It is expected that for patients in groups 2 and 3, factor IX antigen will become detectable in the plasma by 7 days following injection, and in the absence of inhibitor formation will reach plateau levels at 30-40 days. Clinical efficacy will be assessed by examining bleeding records and factor concentrate use at three month intervals during the study and comparing these to information obtained historically for six months prior to enrollment in the trial. In addition, study subjects will be monitored periodically for the presence of vector in blood, saliva, stool, urine and semen until 3 consecutive samples are negative using PCR assay specific for AAV-hFIX sequences. Based on experience with the large animal model, it is expected that vector will likely be detected in serum (and perhaps weakly in other fluids), but for no longer than one day following the injections.

Table III. Inclusion and exclusion criteria

Inclusion Criteria

Males with severe hemophilia B with factor IX activity level <1% of normal

Life expectancy of ≥1 year and ≤20 years

Age ≥18 years old

Ability to give informed consent

Greater than twenty exposure days of treatment with factor IX protein

No history or presence of an inhibitor to factor IX protein

Subjects must be able to infuse factor IX protein on a home infusion protocol

Subjects must be willing to practice barrier birth control until three consecutive semen samples are negative for AAV vector DNA.

Exclusion Criteria

Active acute infections

End stage renal disease

Severe liver disease defined as:

a) Bilirubin: 2.1-3.0 x normal

b) Transaminases: 5-10 x normal

c) Alkaline phosphatase: 5-10 x normal

Platelet count <50,000/μL

Presence of inflammatory muscle disease (*i.e.*, myositis)

Patients who must remain on, or are unwilling to stop, a regimen of prophylactic infusion of factor IX protein

Aside from the discomfort of frequent follow-up visits, specimen collection, muscle biopsy and those associated with intramuscular injection, the risks to patients participating in this trial are largely theoretical ones and center on the potential for integration of vector sequences into chromosomal DNA. Oncogenic transformation of cells due to the insertion of vector sequences into the host cell genome is a theoretical concern, however tumor formation has not been observed in ongoing clinical trials employing vectors that are known to integrate, *e.g.*, retroviral vectors. To date there has been no direct evidence that AAV vector integrates into genomic DNA in skeletal muscle. Dissemination of vector to the gonads and inadvertent transduction of germline tissue is undesirable in a clinical gene transfer protocol. Again, there is no direct evidence that AAV vector integrates into genomic DNA in germline tissue. Animal studies on AAV-mediated transduction of germline tissue following intramuscular injection are nearing completion and suggest that the potential for untoward effects due to the presence of vector sequences in sperm DNA (if any) is 6-7 orders of magnitude less than that observed due to natural transposable elements present in the human genome (27). The clinical trial is designed to minimize both of these theoretical risks by using ultrasound guidance of injections to prevent vector dissemination from muscle and by choosing a muscle that can be completely resected if necessary.

Of more concern is the potential for the development of an inhibitory antibody to factor IX. The average number of days of exposure to clotting factor concentrate prior to the development of inhibitory antibodies in patients at risk is between 10-20 days (23, 25). All subjects in the Phase I/II study will be adults who have severe factor IX deficiency, therefore each subject will have had many more than 20 exposure days to factor IX concentrate. As a further measure of safety, the clinical study has been designed to exclude patients who have any history of inhibitor formation. In addition, the observation that the single dog that produced an inhibitor also had a concomitant skin infection has prompted us to exclude any subject with an active acute infection. It should be pointed out, however, that experience with human trials will be necessary in order to assess the risk of inhibitor formation in the setting of endogenous factor production.

If, as expected, the ongoing Phase I/II clinical study documents the safety of the AAV-mediated muscle-directed gene transfer approach, it will form the basis for later trials aimed at improving the levels of biologically active factor IX protein in patients with hemophilia B. In addition, such experience will pave the way for studies of gene transfer into liver using an AAV vector. Given the very encouraging efficacy data in the dog model of hemophilia B, the potential exists for meaningful increases in plasma levels of factor IX in patients enrolled in the higher dose groups in the Phase I/II trial. If sustained plasma levels of biologically active factor IX similar to those seen in the animal models (50-100 ng/mL representing levels that are 1-2% of normal) are observed in humans, then at these doses, a change in phenotype from severe to moderate or mild may be observed. This would represent the first gene transfer-mediated long-term correction of an inherited disorder due to a single gene defect.

REFERENCES

1. Eyster ME, Gill FM, Blatt PM, Hilgartner MW, Ballard JO and Kinney TR. Central nervous system bleeding in hemophiliacs. Blood **51**:1179-1188, 1978.

2. Andes WA, Wulff K and Smith WB. Head trauma in hemophilia: a prospective study. Arch Int Med **144**:1981-1983, 1984.

3. Bray GL and Lubahn NL. Hemophilia presenting with intracranial hemorrhage. An approach to the infant with intracranial bleeding and coagulopathy. Amer J Dis Child **141**:1215-1217, 1987.

4. Lofqvist T, Nilsson IM, Berntorp E and Pettersson H. Haemophilia prophylaxis in young patients--a long-term follow-up. Journal of Internal Medicine **241**:395-400, 1997.

5. Ljung RCR. Annotation. Can haemophilic arthropathy be prevented? Brit J Haematol **101**:215-219, 1998.

6. Lyon DJ, Chapman CS, Martin C, Brown KE, Clewley JP, Flower AJE and Mitchell VE. Symptomatic parvovirus B19 infection and heat-treated factor IX concentrate. (letter). Lancet **1**:1985, 1989.

7. Laurian Y, Dussaix E, Parquet A, Chalvon-Demersay A, d'Oiron R and Tchernia G. Transmission of human parvovirus B19 by plasma derived factor VIII concentrates. Nouv Rev Fr Haematol **36**:449-453, 1994.

8. Santagostino E, Mannucci PM, Gringeri A and al. e. Transmission of parvovirus B19 by coagulation factor concentrates exposed to 100°C heat after lyophilization. Transfusion **37**:517-522, 1997.

9. Linnen J, Wages Jr. J, Zhang-Keck Z-Y, Fry K, Krawczynski K, Alter H, Koonin E, Gallagher M, Alter M, Hadziyannis S, Karayiannis P, Fung K, Nakatsuji Y, Shih JW-K, Young L, Piatak Jr. M, Hoover C, Fernandez J, Chen S, Zou J-C, Morris T, Hyams K, Ismay S, Lifson J, Hess G, Foung S, Thomas H, Bradley D, Margolis H and Kim J. Molecular cloning and disease association of hepatitis G virus: A transfusion-transmissible agent. Science **271**:505-508, 1996.

10. Naoumov NV, Petrova EP, Thomas MG and Williams R. Presence of a newly described human DNA virus (TTV) in patients with liver disease. Lancet **352**:195-197, 1998.

11. Snyder E and Lipton K. Association Bulletin 94-4--Hepatitis G virus: status report and assessment of clinical relevance. AABB News Briefs **August 1998**:20-21, 1998.

12. Evans JP, Brinkhous KM, Brayer GD, Reisner HW and High KA. Canine hemophilia B resulting from a point mutation with unusual consequences. Proc Natl Acad Sci USA **86**:10095-10099, 1989.

13. Cameron C, Notley C, Hoyle S, McGlynn L, Hough C, Kamisue S, Giles A and Lillicrap D. The canine factor VIII cDNA and 5' flanking sequence. Thromb Haemost **79**:317-322, 1998.

14. Bi L, Lawler AM, Antonarakis SE, High KA, Gearhart JD and Kazazian HH. Targeted disruption of the mouse factor VIII gene: A model for hemophilia A. Nature Genet. **10**:119-121, 1995.

15. Lin H-F, Maeda N, Smithies O, Straight DL and Stafford DW. A coagulation factor IX-deficient mouse model for human hemophilia B. Blood **90**:3962-3966, 1997.

16. Snyder R, Xiao X and Samulski R. Production of recombinant adeno-associated viral vectors in N. e. a. Dracopoli. Current Protocols in Human Genetics. New York, John Wiley & Sons. 1-24. 1996.

17. Kaplitt MG, Leone R, Samulski RJ, Xiao X, Pfaff DW, O'Malley KL and During MJ. Long-term expression and phenotypic correction using adeno-associated virus vectors in the mammalian brain. Nature Genet **8**:148-154, 1994.

18. Kessler PD, Podsakoff GM, Chen X, McQuiston SA, Colosi PC, Matelis LA, Kurtzman GJ and Bryne BJ. Gene delivery to skeletal muscle results in sustained expression and systemic delivery of a therapeutic protein. Proc Natl Acad Sci USA **93**:14082-14087, 1996.

19. Herzog R, Yang E, Couto L, Hagstrom J, Elwell D, Fields P, Burton M, Bellinger D, Read M, Brinkhous K, Podsakoff G, Nichols T, Kurtzman G and High K. Long-term correction of canine hemophilia B by gene transfer of blood coagulation factor IX mediated by adeno-associated viral vector. Nature Medicine **5**:56-63, 1999.

20. Tawa N and Goldberg A. Myology. New York, McGraw-Hill, Inc. 1994.

21. Lusher JM, Arkin S, Abildgaard CF and Schwartz RS. Recombinant factor VIII for the treatment of previously untreated patients with hemophilia A. New Engl J Med **328**:453-459, 1993.

22. Bray GL, Gomperts ED, Courter S, Gruppo R, Gordon EM, Manco-Johnson M, Shapiro A, Scheibel E, White G and Lee M. A multicenter study of recombinant factor VIII (recombinate): Safety, efficacy, and inhibitor risk in previously untreated patients with hemophilia A. Blood **83**:2428-2435, 1994.

23. Schwarzinger I, Pabinger I, Korninger C, Haschke F, Kundi M, Neissner H and Lechner K. Incidence of inhibitors in patients with severe and moderate hemophilia A treated with factor VIII concentrates. Am J Hematol **24**:241, 1987.

24. Rasi V and Ikkala E. Haemophiliacs with factor VIII inhibitors in Finland: Prevalence, incidence and outcome. Brit J Haematol **76**:369, 1990.

25. Ehrenforth S, Kreuz W, Scharrer I, Linde R, Fund M, Gungor T, Krackhardt B and Kornhuber B. Incidence of development of factor VIII and factor IX inhibitors in haemophiliacs. Lancet **339**:594, 1992.

26. Hoyer LW. The incidence of factor VIII inhibitors in patients with severe hemophilia A. Adv Exper Med & Biol **386**:35-46, 1995.

27. Kazazian HH. An estimated frequency of endogenous insertional mutations in humans. Nat Genet **22**:130, 1999.

5

USE OF PROPHYLAXIS TO PREVENT COMPLICATIONS OF HEMOPHILIA

P.M. Mannucci, L. Mendolicchio, A.Gringeri
Angelo Bianchi Bonomi Hemophilia and Thrombosis Center, IRCCS
Maggiore Hospital and University of Milan, Italy

The main principle of treatment of hemophilia is the replacement of the deficient coagulation factor with plasma-derived or recombinant products. The goal of replacement therapy may be either the prompt arrest of bleeding (episodic or on demand treatment) or its prevention through the regular administration of factor (prophylaxis).

At the moment, replacement therapy is given only on the occasion of bleeding episodes in the majority of treatment centers throughout the world. Even though such on demand treatment cannot prevent the development of some degree of joint damage [1], many consider it satisfactory, particularly after home infusion has substantially reduced the time interval between the onset of bleeding and replacement therapy. Since the late 1950s Swedish investigators did evaluate the feasibility and efficacy of prophylactic treatment, based upon regularly spaced factor infusions irrespective of the occurrence of bleeding [2]. The rationale for this mode of treatment delivery was offered by the natural history of hemophilia. Hemophiliacs with moderately severe disease, with factor levels measurable at 1-2%, usually do not develop severe musculoskeletal damage and the corresponding handicaps typical of patients with severe hemophilia who have unmeasurable factor levels (<1%) [3]. The idea was that of using prophylaxis to transform severe into moderately severe hemophiliacs and thereby to prevent the main complication of the disease.

THE DEVELOPMENT OF PROPHYLAXIS IN SWEDEN

In Sweden, prophylactic treatment has developed over three decades. In the early periods, limited availability of anti-hemophilic products led to suboptimal dosages and large between-treatment intervals. The intervals between factor infusions, usually given at doses of 10 to 20 IU/kg body weight, were sometime as long as 4 to 10 days [2]. With such large intervals between infusions, plasma factor VIII or IX levels were unmeasurable for prolonged period of times, so that breakthrough bleeding and the resulting musculoskeletal damage could not be completely prevented. In addition, most patients were started on prophylaxis when they had bled on multiple occasions and had already developed some degree of joint damage. As it could be expected prophylaxis carried out according to these early and inadequate protocols did not stop further deterioration of damaged joints. However, it was observed that development of new damage was prevented in those few patients who began treatment at a time when there was no or little damage [2]. These results convinced the Swedish investigators that prophylaxis should be started at a very early age (between one and two years).

In the last fifteen years, these early observations and the increased availability of larger amounts of anti-hemophilic products led to the development of newer prophylaxis schedules that aim to achieve the almost total prevention of bleeding [4,5]. Prophylactic treatment now starts in Sweden when hemophilic boys are one to two years old, preferably when no joint bleeding has yet occurred, and continues until they are at least twenty or older. The schedule currently recommended to patients with severe hemophilia A is based upon the administration every other day of 25 to 40 IU/kg of factor VIII, or of the factor doses needed by each patient to have trough plasma levels no lower than 1% [4,5]. For hemophilia B, the longer half-life of factor IX permits twice weekly infusions of the same dosages. Factors are given at home through peripheral veins, even though central venous lines are needed in several instances in younger children [6,7]. The placement of such central lines is not without problems, because infectious complications develop in a number of patients [6,7].

The overall efficacy of prophylaxis has recently been re-evaluated in Sweden [4,5,8,9]. Patients who were enrolled in the early period, started on prophylaxis at a relatively advanced age when several joint bleeds had already occurred and were treated with suboptimal doses at large intervals, developed clinical and radiological signs of joint involvement. Conversely, patients started on prophylaxis at a very young age before the onset of any bleeding episode and treated with larger and less spaced doses, had little or no clinical and radiological sign of joint damage [8,9].

USE OF PROPHYLAXIS IN OTHER COUNTRIES

Notwithstanding the uncontrolled and retrospective design of the studies carried out in Sweden, several national and international groups have adopted prophylaxis as the method of choice for treatment delivery in hemophiliacs. Recommendations for prophylaxis have been issued in a joint document by the World Health Organization and the World Federation of Hemophilia in 1994, followed in the same year by the United Kingdom Hemophilia Center Directors' Organization, the Association of Hemophilia Clinic Directors of Canada in 1995 and the Netherlands Hemophilia

Treaters in 1996 [10-13]. These recommendations stem from the results of several small non-randomized trials carried out in different countries and of a large one, the Orthopedic Outcome Study [1]. Although not randomized and uncontrolled, this study has provided the most convincing data in support of the results of the Swedish studies. The Orthopedic Outcome Study was a prospective study meant to evaluate whether or not increasing factor utilization decreases the amount of joint damage. In the frame of this study, which enrolled 447 patients with a wide range of joint damage, there was a subset of patients who at entry in the study had normal joints both clinically and radiologically. At the end of the study, 6 years later, half of these children still had normal joints. When children who maintained normal joints were compared with those whose joints deteriorated, it was noticed that the former used larger amounts of factors and were more often treated prophylactically than the latter. Therefore, the study concluded that prophylaxis given at a very early patient age reduces the rate at which joints degenerate, both clinically and radiologically.

That prophylaxis is more efficacious than on demand therapy in preventing hemophilic arthropathy is plausible not only on the basis of these results but simply on the basis of common sense and of our knowledge of the natural history of hemophilia. Yet, prophylaxis is very expensive and evidence of cost-effectiveness is meager [14-16] There are other considerations that cast doubts on the target "prophylaxis for all in the new millennium." At least 10-15% of patients with factor levels below 1% rarely bleed spontaneously and have no joint damage [1]. These "mild-severe" hemophiliacs, who cannot be easily recognized with clinical or laboratory markers, would be submitted to unnecessary infusions and cause unnecessary costs. In addition, the widespread and disciplined acceptance by Swedish hemophiliacs and their families of the burden of repeated intravenous infusions and of the likely application of a central venous line may not be applicable to all communities of hemophiliacs. We have observed that when a boy is born with hemophilia within families who had previous cases and have witnessed the dramatic improvement in the quality of life brought about by on demand home infusion, there is sometime reluctance to embark in such a demanding program as prophylaxis. Finally, many National Health Services and third-party payers are not willing to reimburse prophylaxis unless a randomized, controlled study demonstrates its superiority to on demand treatment in terms of cost, effectiveness, and acceptability.

ONGOING RANDOMIZED STUDIES

There are no randomized prospective studies of prophylaxis. Most of the studies have compared individuals of different ages, over time, at individual centers. The only way to solve the doubts that surround the use of prophylaxis as the main mode of treatment delivery in hemophilia and to convince health authorities to fund this treatment is to carry out prospective, randomized clinical trials comparing efficacy, cost and feasibility of prophylaxis versus on demand treatment. Two studies of this type are now in progress in Italy and the USA. Evaluation Study on Prophylaxis: a Randomized Italian Trial (ESPRIT) is a prospective randomized, open-label comparative study designed to evaluate the efficacy of primary prophylaxis in preventing joint damage and in reducing the frequency of bleeding. The risk of development of factor VIII inhibitors, feasibility and costs in comparison with "on demand" treatment are also evaluated. Forty-five severe hemophilia A patients (factor VIII levels less than 1%) without inhibitors, aged less than 7 years, with negative clinical-radiological joint score at entry and at least one bleeding episode during the last 6 months were enrolled in the study. Until now, 21 patients (median age: 4.0 years, range 9 months –7 years) have been randomized to prophylaxis with recombinant factor VIII, given at a dosage of 25 IU/kg three times a week (Recombinate®).In the early phase of the study, factor VIII assays are carried out before each infusion to evaluate whether or not the goal of avoiding trough factor levels below 1% is achieved. Nineteen patients (median age: 3.8 years, range 1-7 years) are randomized to "on demand" treatment with doses of at least 25 IU/kg that can be repeated as judged necessary by the physician in charge until resolution of the episode is complete. Only very preliminary results are available after two years of follow-up. Two patients randomized to prophylaxis and three randomized to on demand treatment withdrew their consent to participate to the trial after they knew the treatment assigned. Eleven of 21 patients assigned to prophylaxis required central venous lines, whereas none of the on-demand patients did. Two of the port-bearing patients had an infectious complication, treated successfully with antibiotics without discontinuation of prophylaxis. Three of 21 prophylaxis patients developed factor VIII inhibitors and were withdrawn from the study. The prophylactic dose of recombinant factor VIII selected for the study (25 IU/kg) was sufficient to maintain factor VIII plasma levels above 1% in all patients, except two who required 30 and 40 IU/kg respectively. 48 breakthrough hemorrhages were reported until now, usually after traumas. Prophylaxis was very well accepted by families and no infusion was missed. On demand treatment patients used a wide range of doses per infusion (1 to 7) for a total of 369 bleeding episodes, one infusion being successful in 73% of cases. Therefore, after 2-years of follow-up, prophylaxis was shown to be safe, highly accepted by families and efficacious in reducing the number of bleeding episodes. The selected prophylactic dose of 25 IU/kg was usually sufficient to prevent bleeding episodes and maintain factor VIII plasma levels above 1%.

The goal of the randomized prospective USA study, which is supported by the Centre for Disease Control and Prevention, is to compare two different treatment arms in small children for the prevention of bleeding and the development of damage in six different index joints: ankles, elbows and knees. Costs and efficacy are also looked at. Complications are evaluated including infections and development of inhibitor, and there is a psycho-social evaluation that will look at quality of life, family coping and child self-esteem. Eligibility for the study includes having a factor VIII activity of less than 2%, being 12 to 30 months of age and not having had more than two bleeds into the same index joint, that must be normal clinically and on X-ray at entry. In the prophylaxis arm of the study, children receive 25 IU/kg of recombinant factor VIII (Kogenate®) every other day. If they have breakthrough bleeds the dose is increased up to a maximum of 35 IU/kg every other day. If a port is needed it is placed and to date 21 of 23 children randomized to prophylaxis needed a port. In the on demand arm, at a time of a joint bleed the child receives 40 IU/kg on the day of the bleed, 20 IU/kg the next day and 20 IU/kg at 72 hours. Further doses can be given at discretion of the treater. Trough factor VIII levels are measured 48 hours after the last infusion, but the information is not used to change the dose. The end point of the study will be when the children are 6 years of age. At the time of writing this chapter, we know that 48 patients have been enrolled in the study and that there was no withdrawal, but data on inhibitor incidence are not available as yet.

The two studies on prophylaxis have similarities and differences. Both are randomized and foresee the same prophylactic dose of factor VIII (25 IU/kg) at intervals of 48 hours. The monitoring plan and end points are also similar. They are somewhat different in the enrollment criteria, in that in the USA study children with severe hemophilia are enrolled at on earlier age, similar to that recommended in Sweden (1 to 2 years), whereas the median age of the Italian patients is higher (4 years). Another substantial difference is the on demand treatment, that is more aggressive in the USA than in the Italian study: initial dose 40 IU/kg versus 25 IU/kg, with two scheduled doses of 20 IU/kg in the next 48 hours which are not part of the Italian schedule. These differences notwithstanding, there are enough similarities in design among the two studies to allow the possibility of merging the results into a metanalysis if the size of each study will turn out to be inadequate.

CONCLUSIONS

The major morbidity of hemophilia is joint damage. Despite their uncontrolled design, the pioneer Swedish studies have convinced the hemophilia community that early prophylaxis can prevent the development of joint damage. Unfortunately, prophylaxis is expensive, about three time more expensive than on demand treatment [14]. In Italy, if we were to begin a child of 1 to 2 years of age on prophylaxis, the expenses at 10 years would be the equivalent of one million dollars. Third-party payers, in our as well as in other countries, look at evidence-based medicine, and prophylaxis cannot be recommended at the moment on these grounds. A substantial saving of money could be accomplished if we could give prophylactic factor VIII by continuous intravenous infusion, but currently available devices are not advanced enough to allow this in the average hemophiliac on treatment at home. If the overall results of the ongoing prophylaxis trials are satisfactory it will perhaps be easier to achieve the goal of putting most children on prophylactic treatment. At the moment, despite the recommendations made by many organizations of consumers and providers, prophylaxis is still a luxury available to a small proportion of fortunate patients.

REFERENCES

1. Nilsson IM, Hedner U, Ahlberg A. Hemophilia prophylaxis in Sweden. Acta Paediat Scand 65: 129-135, 1976.

2. Ahlberg A. Haemophilia in Sweden. VII. Incidence, treatment and prophylaxis of arthropathy and other musculo-skeletal manifestations of haemophlia A and B. Acta Orthop Scand 77: 1-98, 1965).

3. Petrini P, Blomback M, Egberg N, Lindvall N. Prophylaxis with factor concentrates in preventing hemophilic arthropathy. Am J Pediat Hematol Oncol 13: 280-287, 1991.

4. Nilsson IM, Berntorp E, Lofquist T, Pettersson H. Twenty-five years' experience of prophylactic treatment in severe haemophilia A and B. J Intern Med 232: 25-32, 1992.

5. Blanchette VS, Al-Musa A, Stain AM, Ingram J, Fille RM. Central venous access devices in children with hemophilia: an up-date. Blood Coag Fibrinol 8: S11-S14, 1997.

6. Ljung R, van den Berg M, Petrini P, Tengborn L, Scheibel E, Kekomaki R, Effenber W. Prot-A-Cath usage in children with haemophilia: experience of 53 cases. Acta Paedit 87:1051-1054, 1998.

7. Lofquist T, Nilsson IM, Berntorp E, Pettersson H. Haemophilia prophylaxis in young patients. A long-term follow-up. J Intern Med 241: 395-400 1997.

8. Berntorp E. Methods of hemophilia care delivery: regular prophylaxis vs. episodic treatment. Haemophilia 1: 3-7, 1995.

9. van den Berg HM, Nieuwenhuis HK, Mauser-Bunchoten EP, Rosendaal G. Haemophilia prophylaxis in the Netherlands. Sem Haematol 31: 13-15 (suppl. 2), 1994.

10. Liesner Rj, Hair K, Hann IM. The impact of prophylactic treatment on children with severe haemophilia. Br J Haem 92: 973-978, 1996.

11. Lusher J. Prophylaxis in children with hemophilia: is it the optimal treatment? Thromb Hemostats 78: 726-729, 1997.

12. Manco-Johnson MJ, Nuss R, Geraghty S, Funk S, Kilcoyne R. Results of secondary prophylaxis in children with severe hemophilia. Am J Hematol 47: 113-117, 1994.

13. Smith PS, Teutsch SM, Schaffer PA, Rolka H, Evatt B. Episodic versus prophylactic infusions for hemophilia A: a cost-effectiveness analysis. J Paediat 129: 424-431, 1996.

14. Szucs TD, Offner A, Schramm W. Socioeconomic impact of haemophilia care: results of a pilot study. Haemophilia 2: 211-217, 1996.

15. Bohm RL, Avorn J, Glynn RJ, Choodnovsky I, Haschemeyer R, Aledort LM. Prophylactic use of factor VIII: an economic evaluation. Thromb Haemostas 79: 932-937, 1998.

6
FACTOR VIII INHIBITORS

Pete Lollar, John F. Healey, Rachel T. Barrow
and Ernest T. Parker
Department of Medicine, Emory University, Atlanta GA 30322

Introduction

The differential diagnosis in the bleeding patient includes inhibitory antibodies to blood coagulation proteins. Factor VIII (fVIII) is the most commonly targeted coagulation protein by the immune system. FVIII inhibitors arise as alloantibodies in transfused hemophiliacs and as autoantibodies in nonhemophiliac populations (1-4). They develop in response to fVIII infusions in approximately 25% of patients with hemophilia A (5). In nonhemophiliacs, fVIII autoantibodies develop in a variety of clinical settings, including the postpartum period, systemic erythematosus, and chronic lymphocytic leukemia. Interestingly, autoantibody patients tend to present with more severe bleeding than hemophilia A patients with a *de novo* inhibitor. In both settings, fVIII inhibitors are polyclonal IgG populations directed against multiple epitopes.

Inhibitors act by interfering with the procoagulant function of fVIII. In proteolytically-activated form participates in blood coagulation by serving as a cofactor for factor IX during the proteolytic activation of factor X. A modification of a standard one-stage activated partial thromboplastin-based fVIII assay called the Bethesda assay is the most widely fVIII inhibitor assay method (6). A sample containing inhibitor, such as a dilution of patient plasma or a purified IgG preparation, is incubated with a source of fVIII and then residual fVIII is measured

Hemophilia Care in the New Millennium, edited by D. Monroe *et al.*
Kluwer Academic/Plenum Publishers, 2001

in a clotting assay. The Bethesda titer is the reciprocal of the dilution of inhibitor that produces 50% inhibition of fVIII activity. When the Bethesda titer in a patient's plasma is less than 5 to 10, increasing the dose of fVIII can frequently provide adequate hemostasis. However, at greater titers alternate strategies are required.

Following the development of methods for the isolation and characterization of fVIII and the cloning of the fVIII cDNA, this empirical description of the fVIII inhibitor problem has evolved to a more rigorous understanding (1). The immune response to fVIII involves antibody production by fVIII-specific B cells in a process that involves T cell help. The latter involves recognition of fVIII-specific peptides by T cell receptors in the context of MHC Class II molecules as described elsewhere in this Symposium. In contrast, antibodies tend to recognize discontinuous sequences on proteins that come together and form part of the surface of a protein.

Mapping fVIII epitopes using hybrid human/porcine fVIII molecules

Our work has been directed toward mapping fVIII B cell epitopes with the ultimate aim of modifying them to make them less well recognized by the immune system and its products thereof. We have used a series of recombinant hybrid human/porcine fVIII molecules as tools for epitope mapping domains (7-9). This strategy is based on the observation that clinically significant inhibitors usually cross-react poorly with porcine fVIII (10-12), which forms the basis for the therapeutic use of porcine fVIII concentrate.

FVIII is a large, approximately 300 kDa multi-domain protein that interacts with several macromolecules, including factor IXa, factor X, phospholipid membranes, activated protein C, thrombin, plasmin, and factor Xa. Its domains are designated NH_2-A1-A2-B-*ap*-A3-C1-C2-COOH(13). It is cleaved intracellularly and circulates as an A1-A2-B/*ap*-A3-C1-C2 heavy chain/light chain heterodimer (14). During proteolytic activation by thrombin, the B domain and 41-residue light chain activation peptide, *ap*, are released and cleavage occurs between the A1 and A2 domains. The final product is a 160 kDa A1/A2/A3-C1-C2 fVIIIa heterotrimer(15,16).

Hybrid fVIII molecules are created by swapping whole or part of porcine domains for the corresponding human domains. The B domain has no known function and can be deleted entirely from recombinant constructs. Additionally, the B domain rarely, if ever, is a target for inhibitors. Therefore, our work has used B-domainless fVIII hybrids for mapping purposes. We have used hybrid molecules that retain procoagulant activity. Therefore, reduction in antigenicity is unlikely to be due to improper folding of the protein. In contrast, epitope localization by deletion mapping is complicated by the possibility that loss of antigenicity can occur by denaturation of the polypeptide chain.

Additionally, to map A2 and C2 epitopes, we have used exceptional patient plasmas that are specific for the A2 or C2 domains. In contrast, antibodies that are specific for domains outside of A2 and C2 are rare (17), which makes mapping epitopes outside this region more difficult.

The A2 Epitope

Anti-A2 inhibitors block fVIIIa function by binding the fVIIIa-factor IXa-phospholipid complex and block factor X activation noncompetitively (18). The A2 epitope has been mapped using hybrid human/porcine fVIII molecules containing various substitutions of porcine fVIII. The most informative of these, called HP9, contains a porcine substitution for residues Arg484-Ile508 (Fig. 1). The antigenicity of HP9 toward several patient A2-specific inhibitors studied was at least ten-fold

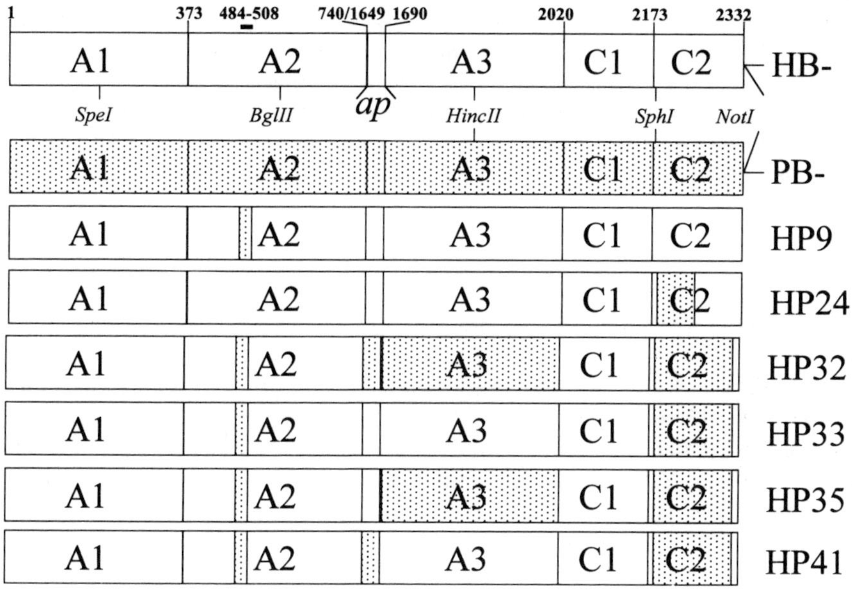

Fig. 1. Hybrid human/porcine fVIII constructs used for epitope mapping. Amino acid numbering refers to mature, full-length human fVIII (45). Human and porcine B-domainless fVIII constructs are designated HB- and PB-, respectively. *Stippled regions* correspond to areas of porcine substitution.

lower than human fVIII (8). This indicates that the segment bounded Arg484-Ile508 contains most, if not all of the binding energy for A2 inhibitors.

The existence of an epitope that can be largely accounted for by a linear sequence is unusual but can occur when the sequence consists of a large loop structure (19,20). There is no X-ray structure available for fVIII. However, modeled structures of the A domains of fVIII exist based on the X-ray structures of nitrite reductase and ceruloplasmin (21,22). Ceruloplasmin is considerably more similar to fVIII than is nitrite reductase. Both proteins have three A domains that are homologous to fVIII and that consist of two plastocyanin-type β-barrel subdomains. The fVIII structures have A1-A2-A3 domains that are arranged in a pseudo-three-fold axis of symmetry. In both structures, the Arg484-Ile508 sequence is a surface exposed loop.

The A2 epitope has been further characterized by making single alanine substitutions at the nine sites the human Arg484-Ile508 region where human and porcine fVIII differ: Arg484, Pro485, Tyr487, Ser488, Arg489, Pro492, Val495, Phe501, and Ile508 (23). The inhibition of these mutants by three A2-specific alloimmune and two A2-specific autoimmune human inhibitor plasmas was measured by the Bethesda assay. For all five patient plasmas, the Tyr487Ala mutant displayed the lowest antigenicity, which ranged from 10 to 20 percent of human fVIII. The inhibition of the Ser488Ala, Arg489Ala, Pro492Ala, Val495Ala, Phe501Ala, and Ile508Ala mutants by most of the plasmas also was significantly reduced. These results indicate that the side chains recognized by A2 inhibitors are similar, despite the differing immune settings that give rise to fVIII alloantibodies and autoantibodies.

The C2 epitope

Anti-C2 inhibitors block the binding of activated fVIII to phospholipid(24). Additionally, they may interfere with von Willebrand factor (vWf) binding, as discussed below. A hybrid fVIII containing a substitution of porcine sequence for Glu2181-Val2243 in the human C2 domain, designated HP24 (Fig. 1), was less antigenic than human factor VIII toward of five C2-specific human antibodies and a murine anti-factor VIII monoclonal antibody, NMC-VIII/5 (9). This defines a factor VIII inhibitor epitope determinant bounded by Glu2181-Val2243 at the NH_2-terminal end of the C2 domain.

However, several lines of evidence indicate that the COOH-terminal end of the C2 domain also participates in antibody binding. Synthetic peptides corresponding to the COOH-terminal 30 amino acids of C2 inhibit the binding of fVIII to phospholipid (25-27). Additionally, NMC-VIII/5 inhibits the binding of fVIII to phospholipid (28) and binds a peptide corresponding to Thr2303-Tyr2332 peptide at the extreme COOH-terminus of fVIII (29).

The C2 domain is also involved in the binding of fVIII to vWf (26,30). vWf and phospholipid compete for binding to fVIII (31-33). Additionally, NMC-VIII-5 inhibits the binding of fVIII to vWf as well as to phospholipid (28). Finally, the Thr2303-Tyr2332 synthetic fVIII peptide inhibits the binding of fVIII to vWf (26). These observations indicate that the C2 domain is structurally and functionally complex. The NH_2-terminal and COOH-terminal sequences of the C2 domain may be juxtaposed in space and form a single epitope. Consistent with this notion, residues Cys2174-Cys2326, which are at opposite ends of the C2 domain, are disulfide bonded (34).

Studies on an inhibitor to the factor V C2 domain have been conducted using hybrid factor V/fVIII proteins that contain substitutions of fVIII in the factor V C2 domain (21). The inhibitor blocked phospholipid binding and was mapped to the NH2-terminal third of the C2 domain. This result is consistent with fVIII inhibitor epitope mapping studies and suggests that the NH_2-terminal region of the C2 domain of both factors V and VIII contains an immunodominant epitope that is important for phospholipid binding.

FVIII inhibitor epitopes outside the A2 and C2 domains

Several studies are consistent with presence in some fVIII inhibitor plasmas of antibodies that bind to the A3 domain and block the binding of fVIIIa to factor IXa. Antibody neutralization studies have identified several inhibitor plasmas in which fVIII light chain more effectively neutralizes a polyclonal inhibitor plasma or IgG preparation better than the C2 domain alone (17). This indicates the presence of at least one epitope in the fVIII light chain (*ap*-A3-C1-C2) outside the C2 domain. Additionally, a recombinant A3-C1 domain polypeptide lacking the *ap* peptide can be immunoprecipitated by most inhibitor IgGs studied to date (35). Three inhibitor IgGs have been identified that are neutralized by a synthetic peptide corresponding to residues 1804-1819 in the A3 domain. This region encompasses a region defined by residues 1811-1819 that constitutes part of the factor IXa binding site (36). Furthermore, patient IgGs have been identified that inhibit the binding of factor IXa to immobilized fVIII light chain (35,37).

Inhibitors specific for epitopes outside the A2 and C2 domains have not been identified. This makes mapping studies using hybrid fVIII molecules difficult. To approach this problem, we have made combinations of substitutions of porcine sequence in the A2, *ap*, A3 and C2 domains of fVIII (Fig. 1). The antigenicity of a quadruply-substituted (A2/*ap*/A3/C2) hybrid, designated HP32, toward 23 high titer inhibitor plasmas was measured and was less than or equal to B-domainless porcine fVIII. This indicates that epitopes recognized by clinically significant inhibitors are largely confined to the A2, *ap*, A3 and C2 regions of fVIII.

To differentiate between inhibitor binding to the *ap* region *versus* the A3 domain, we constructed two triply-substituted hybrids, HP35 and HP41, that differ from HP32 by containing the human *ap* or human A3 domain, respectively. In four of five plasmas in antibodies had been identified against the *ap*-A3 region, the cross-reactivity of HP35 was greater than HP32 and the cross-reactivity of HP41 was less than HP33, which contains porcine substitutions in A2 and C2. This identifies an additional inhibitory epitope in the *ap* peptide of fVIII.

When fVIII is proteolytically activated, the *ap* peptide is released (38). This step is necessary for fVIII to dissociate from von Willebrand factor and participate in blood coagulation (39,40). Thus, antibodies to the *ap* segment may block the activation of the fVIII-von Willebrand factor complex.

Therapeutic implications

Porcine fVIII concentrate (HYATE:C) is useful in inhibitor patients who do not have significant cross-reactivity with porcine fVIII (41-43). Some of these patients develop anti-porcine fVIII antibodies. The epitopes recognized by these antibodies have not been characterized in detail. Western blotting has identified anti-porcine antibodies specific for the A1 domain (44), which is rarely targeted by anti-human fVIII antibodies. A hybrid human/porcine fVIII molecule could be superior to porcine fVIII therapeutically if it lacks immunogenic porcine epitopes.

The prevention of inhibitors in patients with hemophilia A is obviously a desirable goal. One way to do this is to create a less immunogenic fVIII molecule. Mapping fVIII epitopes followed by the identification and mutagenesis of immunodominant amino acid side chains is potential way to accomplish this objective.

References

1. Hoyer, L.W. and D. Scandella. 1994. Factor VIII inhibitors: structure and function in autoantibody and hemophilia A patients. *Semin.Hematol.* 31:1-5.

2. Scandella, D., C. Kessler, P. Esmon, D. Hurst, S. Courter, E. Gomperts, M. Felch, and R. Prescott. 1995. Epitope specificity and functional characterization of factor VIII inhibitors. *Advances in Experimental Medicine & Biology* 386:47-63.

3. Scandella, D. 1996. Human anti-factor VIII antibodies: epitope localization and inhibitory function. *Vox Sanguinis* 70 Suppl 1:9-14.

4. Lollar, P. 1997. Analysis of factor VIII inhibitors using hybrid human/porcine factor VIII. *Thromb.Haemostas.* 78:647-651.

5. Lusher, J.M., S. Arkin, C.F. Abildgaard, R.S. Schwartz, and Kogenate Previously Untreated Patient Study Group. 1993. Recombinant factor VIII for the treatment of previously untreated patients with hemophilia A. Safety, efficacy, and the development of inhibitors. *N.Engl.J.Med.* 328:453-459.

6. Kasper, C.K., L.M. Aledort, R.B. Counts, J.R. Edson, J. Frantatoni, D. Gree, J.W. Hampton, M.W. Hilgartner, J. Lazerson, P.H. Levine, C.W. McMillan, J.G. Pool, S.S. Shapiro, N.R. Shulman, and J. van Eyes. 1975. A more uniform measurement of factor VIII inhibitors. *Thromb.Diath.Haemorrh.* 34:869-872.

7. Lubin, I.M., J.F. Healey, D. Scandella, M.S. Runge, and P. Lollar. 1994. Elimination of a major inhibitor epitope in factor VIII. *J.Biol.Chem.* 269:8639-8641.

8. Healey, J.F., I.M. Lubin, H. Nakai, E.L. Saenko, L.W. Hoyer, D. Scandella, and P. Lollar. 1995. Residues 484-508 contain a major determinant of the inhibitory epitope in the A2 domain of human factor VIII. *J.Biol.Chem.* 270:14505-14509.

9. Healey, J.F., R.T. Barrow, H.M. Tamim, I.M. Lubin, M. Shima, D. Scandella, and P. Lollar. 1998. Residues Glu2181-Val2243 contain a major determinant of the inhibitory epitope in the C2 domain of human factor VIII. *Blood* 92:3701-3709.

10. Morrison, A.E., C.A. Ludlam, and C. Kessler. 1993. Use of porcine factor VIII in the treatment of patients with acquired hemophilia. *Blood* 81:1513-1520.

11. Fiks-Sigaud, M., L. Bendelac, A. Parquet, G. Verroust, M.F. Torchet, A.M. Berthier, E. Fressinaud, C. Guerios, M.F. Aillaud, B. Boneu, A. Derlon, E. Subtil, M.A. Bertrand, J.Y. Borg, and Y. Laurian. 1993. Comparison of anti-human and anti-porcine factor VIII inhibitor levels in 63 patients with severe hemophilia A. *Vox Sang.* 64:210-214.

12. Lloyd, J.V., A.M. Street, E. Berry, J. McPherson, H. Ekert, A. Lammi, McWhirter, WR, E.M. Duncan, E.L. Maxwell, J. Rowell, R.I. Baker, M.F. Leahy, and D. Jupe. 1997. Cross-reactivity to porcine factor VIII of factor VIII inhibitors in patients with haemophilia in Australia and New Zealand. *Australian & New Zealand Journal of Medicine* 27:658-664.

13. Vehar, G.A., B. Keyt, D. Eaton, H. Rodriguez, D.P. O'Brien, F. Rotblat, H. Oppermann, R. Keck, W.I. Wood, R.N. Harkins, E.G.D. Tuddenham, R.M. Lawn, and D.J. Capon. 1984. Structure of human factor VIII. *Nature* 312:337-342.

14. Fass, D.N., G.J. Knutson, and J.A. Katzmann. 1982. Monoclonal antibodies to porcine factor VIII coagulant and their use in the isolation of active coagulant protein. *Blood* 59:594-600.

15. Lollar, P. and C.G. Parker. 1989. Subunit structure of thrombin-activated porcine factor VIII. *Biochemistry* 28:666-674.

16. Curtis, J.E., S.L. Helgerson, E.T. Parker, and P. Lollar. 1994. Isolation and characterization of thrombin-activated human factor VIII. *J.Biol.Chem.* 269:6246-6251.

17. Prescott, R., H. Nakai, E.L. Saenko, I. Scharrer, I.M. Nilsson, J. Humphries, D. Hurst, G. Bray, D. Scandella, and Recombinate and Kogenate Study Groups. 1997. The inhibitory antibody response is more complex in hemophilia A patients than in most nonhemophiliacs with fVIII autoantibodies. *Blood* 89:3663-3671.

18. Lollar, P., E.T. Parker, J.E. Curtis, S.L. Helgerson, L.W. Hoyer, M.E. Scott, and D. Scandella. 1994. Inhibition of human factor VIIIa by anti-A2 subunit antibodies. *J.Clin.Invest.* 93:2497-2504.

19. Laver, W.G., G.M. Air, R.G. Webster, and S.J. Smith-Gill. 1990. Epitopes on protein antigens: misconceptions and realities. *Cell* 61:553-556.

20. Jin, L., B.M. Fendly, and J.A. Wells. 1992. High resolution functional analysis of antibody-antigen interactions. *J.Mol.Biol.* 226:851-865.

21. Ortel, T.L., M.A. Quinn-Allen, F.G. Keller, J.A. Peterson, D. Larocca, and W.H. Kane. 1994. Localization of functionally important epitopes within the second C-type domain of coagulation factor V using recombinant chimeras. *J.Biol.Chem.* 269:15898-15905.

22. Pemberton, S., P. Lindley, V. Zaitsev, G. Card, E.G.D. Tuddenham, and G. Kemball-Cook. 1997. A molecular model for the triplicated A domains of human factor VIII based on the crystal structure of human caeruloplasmin. *Blood* 89:2413-2421.

23. Lubin, I.M., J.F. Healey, D. Scandella, and P. Lollar. 1997. Analysis of the human factor VIII A2 inhibitor epitope by alanine scanning mutagenesis. *J.Biol.Chem.* 272:30191-30195.

24. Arai, M., D. Scandella, and L.W. Hoyer. 1989. Molecular basis of factor-VIII inhibition by human antibodies - antibodies that bind to the factor-VIII light chain prevent the interaction of factor-VIII with phospholipid. *J.Clin.Invest.* 83:1978-1984.

25. Foster, P.A., C.A. Fulcher, R.A. Houghten, and T.S. Zimmerman. 1990. Synthetic factor VIII peptides with amino acid sequences contained within the C2 domain of factor VIII inhibit factor VIII binding to phosphatidylserine. *Blood* 75:1999-2004.

26. Saenko, E.L., M. Shima, K.J. Rajalakshmi, and D. Scandella. 1994. A role for the C2 domain of factor binding to von Willebrand factor. *J.Biol.Chem.* 269:11601-11605.

27. Gilbert, G.E. and J.D. Baleja. 1995. Membrane-binding peptide from the C2 domain of factor VIII forms an amphipathic structure as determined by NMR spectroscopy. *Biochemistry* 34:3022-3031.

28. Shima, M., D. Scandella, A. Yoshioka, H. Nakai, I. Tanaka, S. Kamisue, S. Terada, and H. Fukui. 1993. A factor VIII neutralizing monoclonal antibody and a human inhibitor alloantibody recognizing epitopes in the C2 domain inhibit binding to von Willebrand factor and to phosphatidylserine. *Thromb.Haemostas.* 69:240-246.

29. Scandella, D., G.E. Gilbert, M. Shima, H. Nakai, C. Eagleson, M. Felch, R. Prescott, K.J. Rajalakshmi, L.W. Hoyer, and E. Saenko. 1995. Some human inhibitor antibodies recognize a common epitope corresponding to C2 domain amino acids 2248-2312 which overlap a phospholipid binding site. *Blood* 86:1811-1819.

30. Saenko, E.L. and D. Scandella. 1997. The acidic region of the factor VIII light chain and the C2 domain together form the high affinity binding site for von Willebrand factor. *J.Biol.Chem.* 272:18007-18014.

31. Lajmanovich, A., G. Hudry-Clergeon, J.M. Freyssinet, and G. Marguerie. 1981. Human Factor VIII procoagulant activity and phospholipid interactions. *Biochim.Biophys.Acta* 678:132-136.

32. Andersson, L.O. and J.E. Brown. 1981. Interaction of Factor VIII-von Willebrand Factor with phospholipid vesicles. *Biochem.J.* 200:161-167.

33. Fay, P.J., J.-V. Coumans, and F.J. Walker. 1991. von Willebrand factor mediates protection of factor VIII from activated protein C-catalyzed inactivation. *J.Biol.Chem.* 266:2172-2177.

34. McMullen, B.A., K. Fujikawa, E.W. Davie, U. Hedner, and M. Ezban. 1995. Locations of disulfide bonds and free cysteines in the heavy and light chains of recombinant human factor VIII (antihemophilic factor A). *Protein Sci.* 4:740-746.

35. Zhong, D., E.L. Saenko, M. Shima, M. Felch, and D. Scandella. 1998. Some human inhibitor antibodies interfere with factor VIII binding to factor IX. *Blood* 92:136-142.

36. Lenting, P.J., J.W. van de Loo, M.J. Donath, J.A. van Mourik, and K. Mertens. 1996. The sequence Glu1811-Lys1818 of human blood coagulation factor VIII comprises a binding site for activated factor IX. *J.Biol.Chem.* 271:1935-1940.

37. Fijnvandraat, K., P.H.N. Celie, E.A.M. Turenhout, J.W. Ten Cate, J.A. van Mourik, K. Mertens, M. Peters, and J. Voorberg. 1998. A human alloantibody interferes with binding of factor IXa to the factor VIII light chain. *Blood* 91:2347-2352.

38. Lollar, P., D.C. Hill-Eubanks, and C.G. Parker. 1988. Association of the factor VIII light chain with von Willebrand factor. *J.Biol.Chem.* 263:10451-10455.

39. Hill-Eubanks, D.C. and P. Lollar. 1990. von Willebrand factor is a cofactor for thrombin-catalyzed cleavage of the factor VIII light chain. *J.Biol.Chem.* 265:17854-17858.

40. Hill-Eubanks, D.C., C.G. Parker, and P. Lollar. 1989. Differential proteolytic activation of factor VIII-von Willebrand factor complex by thrombin. *Proc.Natl.Acad.Sci.USA* 86:6508-6512.

41. Kernoff, P.B.A. 1984. Porcine factor VIII: preparation and use in treatment of inhibitor patients. In Factor VIII Inhibitors. L.W. Hoyer, editor. Alan R. Liss, New York. 207-224.

42. Brettler, D.M. 1996. Inhibitors in congenital haemophilia. *Bailliere's Clinical Haematology* 9:319-329.

43. Cohen, A.J. and C.M. Kessler. 1996. Acquired inhibitors. *Bailliere's Clinical Haematology* 9:331-354.

44. Koshihara, K., J. Qian, P. Lollar, and L.W. Hoyer. 1995. Immunoblot crossreactivity of factor VIII inhibitors with porcine factor VIII. *Blood* 86:2183-2190.

45. Wood, W.I., D.J. Capon, C.C. Simonsen, D.L. Eaton, J. Gitschier, B. Keyt, P.H. Seeburg, D.H. Smith, P. Hollingshead, K.L. Wion, E. Delwart, E.G.D. Tuddenham, G.A. Vehar, and R.M. Lawn. 1984. Expression of active human factor VIII from recombinant DNA clones. *Nature* 312:330-337.

7
USE OF HIGH DOSE FACTOR VIIa IN HEMOPHILIA PATIENTS

Ulla Hedner, M.D.
Novo Nordisk, A/S, Målov, Denmark
University of Lund, Lund, Sweden

Background

Hemophilia patients with high titer inhibitors against FVIII/FIX do not benefit from the administration of FVIII/FIX concentration unless special measures to overcome or to remove the inhibitors are undertaken. None of these procedures are easy to perform and cannot be used in acute bleeds or in moderate to mild joint or muscle bleedings. Porcine FVIII may be efficient in patients with non cross-reacting antibodies against FVIII, but do not provide hemostasis in hemophilia B patients with inhibitors against FIX (Macik 1993; Brettler et al. 1989). The hemostatic effect of so-called "FVIII By-passing agents", activated prothrombin complex concentrates (APCC) in serious, life-threatening bleedings and major surgery is still disputed (Macik 1993, Lusher et al. 1983, Sjamsoedin et al. 1981).

Factor VIIa occurs in the normal circulation in a concentration corresponding to around 1% of the total FVII protein mass. In normal individuals levels of about 4 ng/ml have been measured and in hemophilia B patients the concentration is close to zero, while the values in hemophilia A patients vary between normal and levels around 50% of the normal (Wildgoose et al. 1992; Morrissey et al. 1993). By increasing the levels of FVIIa in hemophilia patients to above the concentrations found in normals, hemostasis was induced in hemophilia patients with inhibitors against FVIII (Hedner and Kisiel 1983). Injection of purified FVIIa did not induce any thrombo-embolic side-effects or any signs of a systematically activated coagulation (Hedner and Kisiel 1983; Hedner et al. 1990).

Recombinant FVIIa (rFVIIa) in hemophilia has been developed and found to induce hemostasis in life- and limb-threatening bleeds and major surgery in hemophilia A and B patients independent of the inhibitor titer. In total, more than 500 patients have been treated and rFVIIa has been administered in more than 2000 bleedings episodes.

Hemophilia Care in the New Millennium, edited by D. Monroe *et al.*
Kluwer Academic/Plenum Publishers, 2001

rFVIIa (NovoSeven) in surgery

The first patient, a hemophilia A patient with inhibitors against FVIII, was treated in March 1988 in Stockholm in association with surgery, an open synovectomy. Based on in vitro experiments and results from injection of rFVIIa in hemophilia dogs, a dose of around 60 µg/mg was chosen. Neither per- nor postoperatively did any bleeding occur. A meticulous mechanical hemostasis was performed during surgery and antifibrinolytic therapy was administered (Hedner et al. 1988).

Following this successful first use of rFVIIa, a number of patients with inhibitors against FVIII/FIX were treated in association with surgery.

In total 103 surgical procedures were covered with rFVIIa in doses between 70 and 120 µg/kg given every 2-3 hrs. Out of these 103 episodes, 21 were major, 57 minor, and 25 dental surgery. Some patients were given adjunctive antifibrinolytic therapy but the majority did not, depending on the tradition of the different hemophilia centers involved with the treatment.

In *major surgery*, the effect of rFVIIa was judged as excellent to effective in 81% (17/21) of the procedures, in 3/21 as partially effective, and in one patient the therapy was reported as ineffective (Table 1). The hemostatic efficacy was graded as *effective* if "adequate hemostasis could be maintained intraoperatively and during the initial 48-hour postoperative period without the use of alternative factor therapy" and *ineffective* if "the intraoperative or postoperative blood loss was either excessive or alternative factor therapy was required to achieve hemostasis". Two of the "partially effective" treatments were performed in patients with extensive, long-standing hernias. Both experienced full intraoperative hemostasis but bled during the first postoperative day due to missed doses and/or prolonged dose intervals. Both were given doses of between 90 (given as one dose initially) and 70 µg/kg from dose number 2. Following this experience the doses were increased to 90 - 100 µg/kg every 2nd hr for 24 hrs and no bleeding occurred in the two following series of major surgery (Ingerslev et al. 1996, 1998).

Table 1

NovoSeven (rFVIIa) in Surgery

		Efficacy		
	N	Exc./Effective	Partial	Ineffective
"Named patient basis"	103			
– major	21	81% (17/21)	3/21	1/21
– minor	57	86% (49/57)		2/57
– dental surgery	25	82% (23/25)		1/25
Ingerslev et al. (1996)	13			
– major	13	12/13 (1 not assessable)		
Ingerslev et al. (1998)	17			
– major	6	6/6		
– minor	11	11/11		

The only patient described as a failure was a patient in the first series, who was subjected to extensive resection of myonecrotic tissue following a spontaneous rupture of an abscess developed as a result of an inadequately treated bleeding in the hip region. This patient experienced initially effective hemostasis, but a couple of hrs into surgery he developed acute proteolysis and died on the second attempt to finalize the surgical procedure. In between, he had experienced full hemostasis on rFVIIa (Stein et al. 1990).

Most patients subjected to *minor surgery* (86%) experienced an effective hemostasis. The one who failed was given rFVIIa in a Ringer lactate continuous infusion (rFVIIa diluted in a large volume) and the one who failed in *dental surgery* was inadequately dosed.

The *major surgery procedures* included herniotomy, traceotomy, labarotomy, synovectomy, skin grafting, fractures in all the series and the *minor surgery procedures* included central line insertions, AV shunts, punctures etc.

A *randomized trial comparing two doses of rFVIIa, 35 and 90 µg/kg,* in hemophilia patients with inhibitors undergoing *surgery* was reported by Shapiro et al. (1998). NovoSeven was given as a bolus initially and then again as bolus at every 2nd hr for the following 48 hrs. Twenty-nine eligible patients entered the study. There were 11 major surgical procedures (five synovectomies, two hip arthroplasties, one knee joint manipulation with release of adhesions, one knee cartilage repair, one bone graft and one laparoscopic renal biopsy). The 18 minor procedures included placement of central venous catheters in eight cases, placement of other venous access devices in nine cases and removal of a Port-a-Cath in one case.

Overall efficacy showed that 23 of the 29 patients successfully completed the study with satisfactory hemostasis. At wound closure all major surgery patients were rated as having satisfactory hemostasis. Five patients were regarded as hemostatic treatment failures requiring extra doses (up to 180 µg/kg) or alternative hemostatic therapy during the postoperative period (between 8 hrs and 19 days). All but one of these patients were in the low-dose group. The only patient with bleeding problems in the high dose group had experienced satisfactory hemostasis until day 7 when he developed hemarthrosis in the operated joint (knee arthroplasty).

There was a statistically significant difference in efficacy from day 3 to day 5 in favor of the high-dose group compared with the low-dose group (Fig. 1). In the major surgery group, there was a clear reduction in the number of days of dosing required and the number of injections given to high-dose patients compared with those receiving the lower dose.

Based on the results from this study the investigators conclude that rFVIIa appears to be an efficacious first-line agent in surgery and the 90 µg/kg dose is more effective for both minor and major procedures (Shapiro et al. 1998).

rFVIIa (NovoSeven) in "life- and limb-threatening bleeds"

Following the first successfully treated hemophilia patient with inhibitor who underwent open synovectomy under the cover of rFVIIa, rFVIIa was being used in

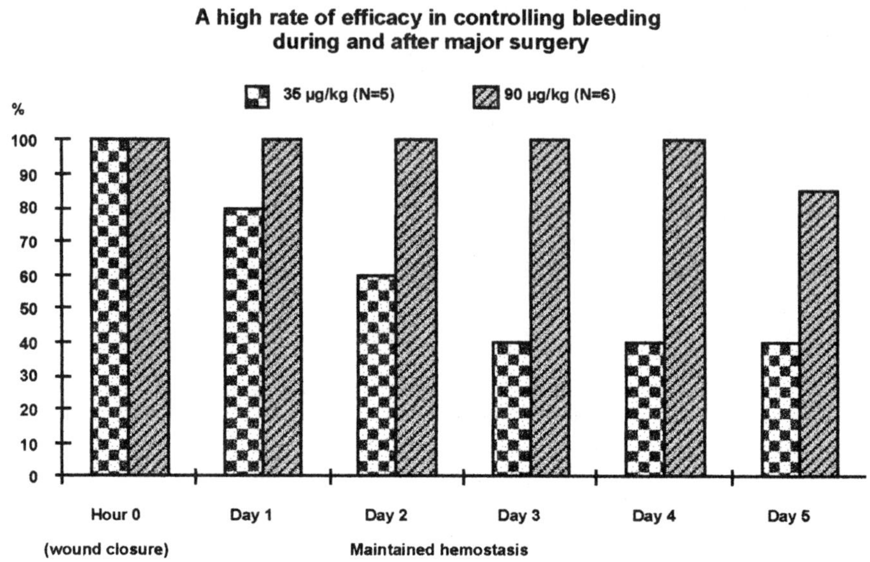

(This figure is based on data from Shapiro et al. 1998)

Fig. 1. The rate of hemostatic efficacy of rFVIIa (NovoSeven) in major surgery comparing two doses, 35 µg/kg and 90 µg/kg given as bolus every 2nd hr. The percentage of efficacy at wound closure, on the first postoperative day (day 1), on day 2, 3, 4, and 5.
The ▣ columns show the result of the low dose of 35 µg/kg and the ▨ columns the result of the higher dose of 90 µg/kg.

an increasing number of emergency situations where all available therapy options (APCC, PCC, porcine FVIII and high doses of FVIII/FIX) already had failed. Patient #2 was treated in Chapel Hill in association with a retropharyngeal hemorrhage (Macik et al. 1989). This program included patients with an acquired inhibitor against FVIII and patients with serious bleeds in the ear, nose and throat region (ENT), the central nervous system (CNS), intra/retroperitoneal and muscle bleeds (compartment syndromes) were treated.

The dose of rFVIIa in most of the patients was 90-100 µg/kg with a range of 60-120 µg/kg given every 2nd hr. The dose intervals following the initial phase and the length of treatment were adjusted to the severity of bleeding and to clinical response.

A computerized algorithm was designed for specific categories of critical bleeds and the overall effective response varied between 62% in muscle bleeds of which several were compartment syndromes and 88% in CNS bleedings (Fig. 2).

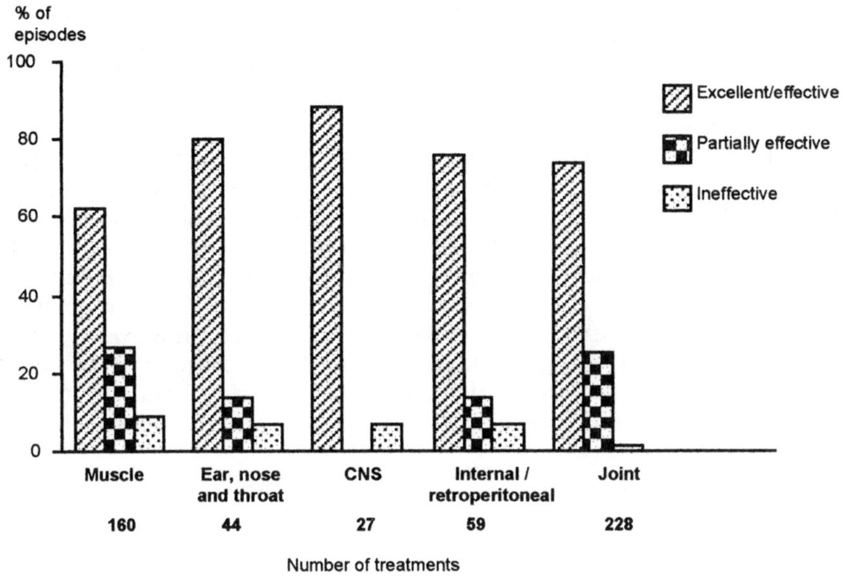

Fig. 2. The hemostatic efficacy of rFVIIa (NovoSeven) in "life- and limb-threatening bleedings" and in fully developed joint bleeds. The serious bleeds are grouped in severe muscle bleeds, ear, nose and throat bleeds, bleedings in the central nervous system (CNS) and in retroperitoneal bleedings. The ▨ columns show the percentage of excellent/effective treatments, the ■ columns the partially effective and the ⛆ columns the ineffective treatments. The number of treatments in each group is given.

rFVIIa (NovoSeven) in mild to moderate bleeds (joint, muscle bleeds)

In a *randomized, double blind, multi-center trial* including 178 *joint, muscle and mucocutaneous bleeding* episodes 78 patients were treated with rFVIIa (35 and 70 µg/kg). In these patients there was a long period of time from onset of bleeding to the start of treatment (8.4 hrs and 10.0 hrs for the lower and higher dose groups, respectively), which most probably contributed to the fact that no significant difference in efficacy between the dose groups was demonstrated. A trend towards a better outcome for joint bleeds treated within 6 hrs was, however, observed (Macik et al. 1993, Lusher et al. 1998). The better effect of early initiated treatment in hemophilia bleedings is well documented and led to the introduction of home treatment in the 1970s. By starting therapy immediately when symptoms appear, the development of full-blown major hemarthrosis is prevented, thereby avoiding the development of synovitis and arthropathy.

To optimize the treatment and to make the treatment situation for the inhibitor patients more similar to hemophilia patients without inhibitors a *home treatment study with rFVIIa was initiated.* A fixed dose of 90 µg/kg at 3 hr intervals within 8 hrs of the onset of a mild to moderate bleeding episode was administered by the patients or their care-givers. After the hemostatic response was rated as "effective" after 1-3 injections, an additional dose of rFVIIa (90 µg/kg) was given 3 hrs later to maintain hemostasis. Thus, for effectively treated bleeds, the number of doses varied from a minimum of two (one treatment plus one maintenance) to a maximum of four (three treatment plus one maintenance). Among the 490 evaluable joint bleeds 452 (92%) were judged as "effective", 24 (5%) as "partially effective" and 8 (2%) as "ineffective. The mean number of injections to achieve hemostasis was among the joint bleeds 2.2 and hemostasis was maintained for at least 24 hrs in 429/452 (95%). Similar results were obtained in the 363 target joints included in the study - 91% rated "effective" and only 2% as ineffective. Maintained hemostasis was seen in 96%. A 92% efficacy and maintenance of 96% was found among the 116 muscle bleeds. The mean time from bleeding to treatment onset was 1.6 hrs for the effectively treated bleeding episodes and 2.4 hrs for those rated as partially effective or ineffective indicating the importance of early start of treatment. Interestingly, a trend towards an improved outcome with increasing number of bleeds was observed (Key et al. 1998).

Adverse Events (AE)

No AE were reported when rFVIIa was used as first line of treatment including home treatment. In total 13 serious AE has been reported, most of which were judged as "non-related" or "most probably non-related" to NovoSeven. In spite of the fact that a number of patients included in the patient group treated in association with life- and limb-threatening bleedings had proven septicemia and a number of the non-hemophilia patients had previously known cardiovascular disease, only one patient developed acute proteolytic activity during extensive surgery including the removal of massive necrotic tissue in the hip region following the spontaneous rupture of an abscess. The consumption in this patient reversed despite continued rFVIIa treatment. According to the physician in charge, rFVIIa was hemostatically effective, and it was considered unclear whether rFVIIa contributed to the condition (Stein et al. 1990).

Several other patients with significant infections or septicemia received treatment with rFVIIa with no signs of consumption coagulopathy. It should also be stressed that another 30 consecutive patients treated for critical bleeds were monitored for changes in D-dimer, antithrombin, α_2-antiplasmin, platelet counts and fibrinogen. No clinically important observations were detected in these assays except for the patient mentioned above (Glazer et al. 1995).

Out of more than 2400 treatment episodes with NovoSeven, two patients developed acute myocardial infarction when on treatment with rFVIIa, one was a 71 year old man with acquired hemophilia and a previous history of diabetes type 2 and cardiovascular disease. The other patient was a heavily overweight hemophilia A patient with inhibitors, 26 yrs old, who had been given massive transfusions, human FVIII, FEIBA, and finally rFVIIa in association with an extensive intraabdominal bleeding bringing him into shock already 2 hrs after the start of bleeding. He recovered without any sequelae.

One 6 yr old hemophilia A boy was given rFVIIa in association with his third CNS bleeding, a left-sided subdural and intraparenchymal hemorrhage. He had severe seizures from the beginning and got large doses of Atavan, phenobarbital and Dilantin. On day 2 he was alert without any neurological symptoms but on day 7 he noticed ataxia. CT scan was negative and rFVIIa and Dilantin were continued. The ataxia improved during the following days and he recovered without any sequelae. It was proposed that the ataxia may have been caused by the high dose of Dilantin given.

No antibodies against rFVIIa have been observed in patients with hemophilia (222 hemophilia A, 16 hemophilia B) with an exposure to rFVIIa between 1 and 121 episodes (Nicolaisen et al. 1996). Furthermore, FVII:C recovery remained unchanged at 6- and 12-month controls of the patients included in the home treatment study suggesting that no neutralizing antibodies to rFVIIa had developed as a result of therapy (Key et al. 1998).

Pharmacokinetic studies were performed in 15 hemophilia patients (10 hemophilia A with inhibitors, four hemophilia A without inhibitors, and one hemophilia B), who all were older than 15 yrs of age. The clearance was found to be 32 ± 8.66 ml/kg/hr and T/2 showed a mean of 2.72 hrs (Lindley et al. 1994). Later, the clearance in 6 hemophilia patients all below 15 yrs of age (three hemophilia A and three hemophilia B), was found to vary between 43.8 and 91.1 ml/kg/hr and their T/2 varied between 1.27 and 1.40 hrs (mean 1.32 hrs) (Hedner et al. 1998).

Mechanism of Action

Hemostasis is initiated by the formation of a complex between tissue factor (TF) and FVII/FVIIa (Rapaport and Rao 1992). TF is normally not exposed to the circulating blood, but is found on a number of various cells in the deeper layers of the vessel wall. TF also has been demonstrated to occur in atherosclerotic plaques and to be expressed by or present within some types of tumor cells. Also, TF has been demonstrated on the surface of monocytes following exposure to bacterial endotoxins as well as after stimulation with growth factors such as platelet-derived factor and monocyte chemotactic protein-1 (Rapaport and Rao 1995; Ernofsson and Siegbahn 1996). Recently it was reported that platelets become TF positive during thrombus formation and it was concluded that blood-borne TF was thrombogenic in an ex vivo model in which human native blood was perfused over collagen-coated slides (Giesen et al. 1999).

Although TF normally is not in contact with circulating blood, FVII and other Vitamin K-dependent coagulation proteins are relatively small proteins and have been demonstrated in the interstitial fluid (Le et al. 1998). TF-FVIIa complexes have been demonstrated to result in some FX activation on the cell surface providing a limited amount of thrombin (Monroe et al. 1997). A certain degree of activation of the hemostasis has been demonstrated in normal individual during normal circumstances as indicated by the presence of both FIX and FX activation peptides in the circulation (Bauer et al. 1990). This process may well be mediated by TF-FVIIa complexes formed in the interstitial tissues while the further propagation of full thrombin generation requires the presence of activated platelets with exposed phosphatidylserine forming the template for binding FIXa (activated by TF-FVIIa), FVIIIa, FVa, and FXa. An interstitial activation of the hemostatic system with the formation of limited amounts of thrombin may thus be the source of the normally occurring activation peptides originating from the activation of

FIX, FX and prothrombin. During normal conditions this may not lead to the deposition of fibrin which is consistent with the report that only negligible amounts of extravascular cross-linked fibrin could be demonstrated in normal guinea pig tissues unless increased vascular permeability was at hand (Dvorak et al. 1985).

Tissue injury or inflammation, by increasing vascular permeability or disrupting endothelial cells could enhance the hemostatic process by exposing TF at the site of injury or increasing the concentration of FVII at the site of TF interstitially.

Such an injury will also increase the availability of platelets and other cells at the site of injury. The platelets will become activated by the thrombin formed initially by the TF-FVIIa complex thereby exposing phosphatidylserine and providing the template for full thrombin generation. This process will still be compartmentalized and confined to the exposed phosphatidylserine and TF. By providing TF-hybrids as described by Giesen et al. (1999) close to the platelet surface the propagation of coagulation in this environment may be facilitated. Although antithrombin does not inhibit free FVIIa, it has been found to inhibit the FVIIa-TF cell surface bound complexes (Rao et al. 1993) indicating an important role of antithrombin in the regulation of the initial FVIIa-TF induced hemostasis.

The administration of exogenous rFVIIa in rather high amounts has been shown to induce hemostasis in patients with hemophilia A and B also in those with inhibitors against FVIII/FIX (Hedner 1990, Glazer et al. 1995). The initial doses used have varied between 70 and 120 μg/kg in most patients. Lower doses have been shown to give a less reliable hemostasis (Gringeri et al. 1991; Shapiro et al. 1998). Using the high doses, rFVIIa induces hemostasis independent of the presence of FVIII/FIX.

Recently, it was shown that higher concentration of FVIIa than what is seen normally in the circulating blood is required to mediate the conversion of FX into FXa independent of TF on a phospholipid surface (Monroe et al. 1997). rFVIIa was found to bind to the activated platelet surface with a low affinity binding. Also, it was demonstrated that thrombin formation in the range of what was seen when normal concentrations of all coagulation proteins were applied to the cell-based system used, was achieved in the absence of FVIII/FIX after addition of rFVIIa concentrations of around or higher than 50 nM. This indicates that rFVIIa in concentrations higher than 50 nM may be able to compensate for the absence of FVIII/FIX, which fits well with the clinical experience of rFVIIa in hemophilia patients with inhibitors against FVIII/FIX. A dose of rFVIIa of around 100 μg/kg (roughly corresponding to a concentration of 50 nM and a FVII:C of 70-90 U/ml) has in those patients shown satisfactory hemostasis in most cases.

However, a substantial variation between individuals regarding the capacity to generate thrombin on the activated platelet surface was demonstrated (Sumner et al. 1996). Accordingly, it may be expected that there will be a substantial variation in the request for rFVIIa in order to normalize the individual full thrombin response in the presence of activated platelets.

In a system containing TF-bearing monocytes, plasma concentrations of the coagulation proteins, inhibitors and unactivated platelets, it was demonstrated that the addition of rFVIIa in increasing concentrations gave a dose-dependent increase in thrombin generation reaching normal level and rate at a concentration of 100 nM of rFVIIa (Kjalke et al. 1999). This may indicate that although a hemostatic effect is being achieved at lower rFVIIa concentrations in most hemophilia patients the effect in terms of a fully normal thrombin generation may require higher doses of rFVIIa. Also, the amount required in each individual may vary substantially as pointed out above.

Thrombin is essential for the formation of a fully stabilized fibrin plug by activating FXIII as well as the "thrombin activated fibrinolytic inhibitor (TAFI) recently described (Bajzar et al. 1995). While FXIII is activated by fairly low concentrations of thrombin (Greenberg et al. 1985), TAFI requires higher concentrations (Bajzar et al. 1995). Since TAFI prevents the conversion of glu-plasminogen into lys-plasminogen thereby down regulating the fibrinolysis, a less than full thrombin burst may result in a defective resistance against fibrinolysis. An increased rate of clot lysis has also been demonstrated in hemophilia patients (Broze and Higuchi 1996). Accordingly, the addition of fibrinolytic inhibitors in the treatment of hemophilia patients especially in association with surgery has been advocated (Nilsson et al. 1977; Ingerslev et al. 1998).

FXI is activated by thrombin and has been demonstrated to enhance the thrombin generation on the activated platelet surface (Oliver et al. 1999). The extra thrombin generated by FXI may be important in providing enough thrombin for the activation of TAFI thereby increasing the resistance against fibrinolysis.

Since FVIIa by itself is enzymatically inactive, the effect of rFVIIa on hemostasis is dependent on the binding of rFVIIa to TF or, in case the rFVIIa concentrations are high enough, phosphatidylserine exposed on the activated platelet surface. The activation of platelets resulting in the exposure of phosphatidylserine is dependent on the initial TF-FVIIa complex formed at the site of exposed TF (Monroe et al. 1997). The normally occurring FVIIa, about 1% of the total FVII protein mass (Wildgoose et al. 1992) may, however, be enough to induce the platelet activation at the site of exposed TF. The TF-FVIIa complexes are then inhibited by the action of TFPI as well as by antithrombin (Rao et al. 1993). Also, the available FVII (10 nM) should be enough to saturate all the TF exposed at the injury site. The hemostatic activity of rFVIIa in high doses seen in hemophilia may primarily be mediated by the binding of rFVIIa to phosphatidylserine exposed on the platelet surface as a result of the activation process provided by the initially TF-FVIIa mediated platelet activation. rFVIIa bound to the platelet surface may on the other hand be inhibited neither by the TFPI nor by antithrombin both requiring the complexes TF-FVIIa for their activity. The compartmentalization of the thrombin generation process seems to be very well regulated by the inhibitor systems as well as the binding capacity of FVIIa to special surfaces. Accordingly, the risk of any development of thromboembolic complications seems to be minimal. However, further studies are needed to elucidate the role of increased levels of FVII in situations with an abundance of TF such as at the time an atherosclerotic plaque undergoes rupture.

Dosing and Administration of NovoSeven

Assuming that a full thrombin burst initially is essential for a full hemostatic effect of rFVIIa, the following key issues in dosing of NovoSeven can be identified

1. *early intervention* is crucial to avoid the development of full blown bleedings that are more difficult to treat (this is no different from hemophilia treatment with FVIII/FIX). In the home treatment study of NovoSeven a mean number of injections of 2.2 was enough to provide hemostasis (Key et al. 1998) as

compared to the more complicated treatments required in patients with compartment syndrome for example (Hedner 1990).
2. *interindividual variation in clearance* has been demonstrated with a substantial difference between patients below or above 15 yrs of age (Lindley et al. 1994; Hedner et al. 1998). The higher clearance rate and the shorter T/2 in individuals below 15 yrs of age should be taken into account when dosing NovoSeven. A higher initial dose may be needed in order to achieve the full thrombin burst in the patients with a higher clearance.
3. *interindividual variation in the capacity of thrombin generation on the surface of activated platelets* has been demonstrated (Sumner et al. 1996). Currently, the thrombin generation in platelet-rich plasma is being studied and hopefully this will lead to the establishment of a method for use in the clinic.

Although doses of 90-120 μg/kg has been shown to be hemostatically effective in most patients, higher doses may give better results keeping the above in mind. The dose of 90-120 μg/kg has to be repeated every 2nd hr initially in case of serious bleedings or surgery. Higher doses of NovoSeven may result in firm, fully stabilized fibrin plugs initially making repeated doses unnecessary.

Continuous infusion. NovoSeven is recommended to be administered as single i.v. bolus injections with a short dose interval of 2 hrs. In case longer intervals had been applied accidentally or by planning, oozing has been observed and in some cases of major surgery also profuse postoperative bleedings occurred. In order to ensure a constant plasma level of FVII:C continuous infusion was introduced by Schulman et al. (1996). Continuous infusion has since long been found convenient and adequate for FVIII as well as FIX-concentrates in the treatment of hemophilia patients (Martinowitz and Schulman 1994). According to the recommendation by Schulman et al. (1996), the maintenance dose of NovoSeven, after the initial bolus dose of 90 μg/kg, should be based on the individual clearance in each patient. Due to changes of the clearance during surgery or treatment, the pharmacokinetics was recommended to be repeated during the treatment and the dose adjusted accordingly (Schulman et al. 1996). In addition, it was also stressed that each pump has to be checked with regard to potential adsorption of rFVIIa to the plastic material. The conclusion drawn by Schulman et al. (1996) was that NovoSeven could be used in continuous infusion provided the pumps were checked as for adsorption of rFVIIa, and that its use added to the convenience and safety of the treatment by avoiding the risk of dangerously low trough levels of FVII:C in plasma due to a delayed or missed injection. Later, however, bleedings have occurred in patients on continuous infusion with NovoSeven. Characteristically, these patients have been strictly given continuous doses of around 15 μg/kg/hr irrespective of the patient's clearance and type of surgery. It seems clear that inadequate dosing of NovoSeven occurred in these patients.

Since the hemostasis induced by exogenous rFVIIa seems to be dependent on a full burst of thrombin generation on the surface of activated platelets, it most probably is important to ensure a dose of exogenous rFVIIa which is high enough to bind to the phosphatidylserine on the activated platelets which means 50 nM or higher. At present it is not known for how long time a concentration of FVII higher than 50 nM would be needed in order to initiate a full, solid hemostasis. Peak values of FVII:C of around or higher than 30 U/ml, however, have been associated with successful hemostasis (Glazer et al. 1995; Shapiro et al. 1998), while failing hemostasis has been observed at trough levels below 10 U/ml (Hedner 1996). A shortening of the prothrombin time (PT) to around 7-8 sec occurs when the FVII:C is 5 U/ml or higher, and can be used to get an arbitrary evaluation of the FVII:C before next dose. In case continuous infusion of rFVIIa is being used, plasma levels of FVII:C at least around 30 to 40 U/ml and preferably peak levels around 50-60 U/ml should be targeted for the first 12 to 24 hrs depending on type of surgery in order to ensure that the concentration of FVIIa is high enough for the required period of time also in individuals with a rapid clearance. This may require doses of 50 up to 120 µg/kg/hr depending on clearance. Depending upon type of surgery this dose may be tapered down to around 15 µg/kg/hr in due time.

Summarizing the experience of NovoSeven administered by continuous infusion, such treatment seems feasible provided that the dose of NovoSeven used is adjusted to each patient's clearance and type of surgery. In addition, the initial bolus dose has to be high enough to peak levels of FVII:C of 50-60 U/ml. It may also be stressed that in order to save a maximum of 25% of drug, one will operate at the lower level of FVII:C necessary for hemostasis making the treatment less robust. This will necessitate a careful monitoring of the patient and daily evaluation of the patient's pharmacokinetics.

In Summary high doses of rFVIIa (NovoSeven) meaning concentrations of at least 50 nM (corresponding to a bolus dose of around 100 µg/kg and FVII:C levels of around 70-90 U/ml) or higher seem to be hemostatically effective and safe in the treatment of patients with inhibitors against FVIII/FIX. One or two doses of rFVIIa may be enough to ensure hemostasis in moderate to mild joint and muscle bleedings when given as an early treatment (home-treatment).

References

Bajzar L, Manuel R, Nesheim ME. Purification and Characterization of TAFI, a Thrombin-activable Fibrinolysis Inhibitor. J Biol Chem 1995;270:14477-84.

Bauer KA, Kass BI, tenCate H Hawiger JJ, Rosenberg RD. Factor IX is activated in vivo by the tissue factor mechanism. Blood 1990;76:731-6.

Brettler DB, Forsberg MS, Levine PH, Aledort LM, Hilgartner M, Kasper CK, Lusher JM, McMillan CW, Roberts H R. The use of porcine factor VIII concentrate (Hyate:C) in the treatment of patients with inhibitor antibodies to factor VIII. A multicenter US experience. Arc Intern Med 1989;149:1381-5.

Broze GJ, Higuchi DA. Coagulation-dependent inhibition of fibrinolysis: role of carboxypeptidase-U and the premature lysis of clots from hemophilic plasma. Blood 1996;88:3815-23.

Dvorak HN, Senger DR, Dvorak AM, Harvey VS, McDonagh J. Regulation of extravascular coagulation by microvascular permeability. Science 1985;227:1059-61.

Ernofsson M, Siegbahn A. Platelet-derived growth factor-BB and monocyte chemotactic protein-1 induce human peripheral blood monocytes to express tissue factor. Thromb Res 1996;83:307-20.

Giesen PLA, Rauch U, Bohrmann B, Kling D, Roque M, Fallon JT, Badimon JJ, Himber J, Riederer MA, Nemerson Y. Blood-borne tissue factor: Another view of thrombosis. Proc Natl Acad Sci USA 1999;96:2311-5.

Glazer S, Hedner U, Falch JF. Clinical update on the use of recombinant factor VIIa. In: Aledort LM, Hoyer LW, Lusher JM, Reisner HM, White II GC (eds): Inhibitors to Coagulation Factors. New York, Plenum Press, 1995; 163-74.

Greenberg CS, Miraglia CC, Rickles FR, Shuman MA. Cleavage of blood coagulation factor XIII and fibrinogen during in vitro clotting. J Clin Invest 1985;75:1463-70.

Gringeri A, Santagostino E, Mannucci PM. Failure of recombinant activated factor VII during surgery on a hemophiliac with high-titer factor VIII antibody. Hemostasis 1991; 21:1-4.

Hedner U, Kisiel W. The use of human factor VIIa in the treatment of two hemophilia patients with high-titer inhibitors. J Clin Invest 1983;71: 1836-41.

Hedner U, Glazer S, Pingel K, Alberts KA, Blombäck M, Schulman S, Johnsson H. Successful use of rFVIIa in a patient with severe haemophilia A subjected to synovectomy. Lancet 1988; ii:1993.

Hedner U, Ljungberg J, Lund-Hansen T. Comparison of the effect of plasma-derived and recombinant human FVIIa in vitro and in a rabbit model. Blood Coag Fibrinolys 1990;1:145-52.

Hedner U. Factor VIIa in the treatment of haemophilia. Blood Coagul Fibrinolysis 1990;1:307-17.

Hedner U. Dosing and monitoring NovoSeven treatment, Haemostasis 26 (suppl 1): 102-108, 1996.

Hedner U, Kristensen HI, Berntorp E, Ljung R, Petrini P. Pharmacokinetics of rFVIIa in children. 23rd International Congress of the World Federation of Hemophilia. The Hague, The Netherlands, May 17-21, 1998.

Ingerslev J, Freidman D, Gastineau D, Gilchrist G, Johnsson H, Lucas G, McPherson J, Preston E, Scheibel E, Schuman M. Major surgery in haemophilic patients with inhibitors using recombinant factor VIIa. Haemostasis 1996; Suppl1:118-23.

Ingerslev J, Sneppen O, Hvid I, Knudsen L, Thykjær H, Fredberg U, Sindet-Petersen S. Experiences with recombinant factor VIIa (rFVIIa) in treatment of haemophilic inhibitor bleeding. In Scharrer I, Schramm W (eds): 27. Hämophilie-Symposion Hamburg 1996; Berlin, Heidelberg 1998, Springer Verlag.

Key NS. Aledort LM, Beardsley D, Cooper H, Davignon D, Ewenstein B, Gilchrist GS, Gill JC, Glader B, Hoots WK, Kisker CT, Lusher JM, Rosenfield CG, Shapiro AD, Smith H, Taft E. Home treatment of mild to moderate bleeding episodes using recombinant factor VIIa (NovoSeven) in haemophiliacs with inhibitors. Thromb Haemost 1998;80:912-8.

Kjalke M, Monroe DM, Hoffman M, Roberts HR, Hedner U, Ezban M. High-dose Factor VIIa restores platelet activation and total thrombin generation in a model system mimicking hemophilia A or B conditions. Int Soc Thromb Haemost Congr, Washington DC, Aug 1999, Abstract.

Le DT, Borgs P, Toneff W, Witte MH, Rapaport SI. Hemostatic factors in rabbit limb lymph: relationship to mechanisms regulating extravascular coagulation. Am J Physiol 1998;274:H769-76.

Lindley CM, Sawyer WT, Macik BG, Lusher J, Harrison JF, Baird-Cox K, Birch K, Glazer S, Roberts HR. Pharmacokinetics and Pharmacodynamics of recombinant factor VIIa. Chir Pharmacol ther, 1994;55:638-44.

Lusher JM, Blatt PM, Penner JA, Aledort LM, Levine PH, White GC, Warrier AI, Whitehurst DA. Autoplex versus Proplex: a controlled, double-blind study of effectiveness in acute hemarthroses in hemophiliacs with inhibitors to factor VIII. Blood 1983;62:1135-8.

Lusher JM, Roberts HR, Dagivnon G, Joist JH, Smith H, Shapiro A, Laurian Y, Kasper CK, Mannucci, PM, and the rFVIIa Study Group. A randomized, double-blind comparison of two dosage levels of recombinant factor VIIa in the treatment of joint, muscle and mucocutaneous haemorrhages in persons with haemophilia A and B, with and without inhibitors. Haemophilia 1998;4:790-8.

Lusher J, Ingerslev J, Roberts H, Hedner U. Clinical experience with recombinant factor VIIa. Blood Coagul Fibrinolysis 1998;9: 119-28.

Macik BG, Lindley CM, Lusher J, Sawyer WT, Bloom AL, Harrison JF, Baird-Cox K, Birch K, Glazer S, Roberts HR. Safety and initial clinical efficacy of three dose levels of recombinant activated factor VIIa (rFVIIa) : results of a Phase I study. Blood Coagul Fibrinolysis 1993;4:521-7.

Macik BG, Hohneker J, Roberts HR, Griffin AM. Use of recombinant activated factor VII for treatment of a retropharyngeal hemorrhage in a hemophilic patient with a high titer inhibitor. Am J Hematol 1989;32:232-4.

Macik BD. Treatment of Factor VIII inhibitors: Products and Strategies. Semin Thromb Hemost 1993;19:13-24.

Martinowitz U, Schulman S. Continuous infusion of coagulation products. Int J Pediatr Hematol Oncol 1994;1:471-8.

Monroe DM, Hoffman M, Oliver JA, Roberts HR. Platelet activity of high-dose factor VIIa is independent of tissue factor. Br J Haematol 1997;99:542-7.

Morrissey JH, Macik BG, Neuenschwander PF, Comp PC. Quantitation of activated factor VII levels in plasma using a tissue factor mutant selectively deficient in promoting factor VII activation. Blood 1993;81:734-44.

Nicolaisen EM, Hansen LL, Poulsen F, Glazer S, Hedner U. Immunological aspects of recombinant factor VIIa (rFVIIa) in clinical use. Thromb Haemost 1996;76:200-4.

Nilsson IM, Hedner U, Ahlberg Å, Larsson SA, Bergentz SE. Surgery of Hemophiliacs - 20 Year's Experience. World J Surg 1977;1:55-68.

Oliver JA, Monroe DM, Roberts HR, Hoffman M. Thrombin Activates Factor XI on Activated Platelets in the Absence of Factor XII. Art Thromb Vasc Biol 1999; 19:170-7.

Rao LVM, Rapaport SI, Hoang AD. Binding of factor VIIa to tissue factor permits rapid antithrombin III/heparin inhibition of factor VIIa. Blood 1993;81:2600-7.

Rapaport SI, Rao LVM. Initiation and regulation of tissue factor-dependent blood coagulation. Art Thromb 1992;12:1111-21.

Rapaport SI, Rao LVM. The tissue factor pathway: how it has become a "prima ballerina". Thromb Haemost 1995;74:7-17.

Schulman S, Bech Jensen M, Varon D, Keller N, Gitel S, Horoszowski H, Heim M, Martinowitz U. Feasibility of using recombinant factor VIIa in continuous infusion. Thromb Haemost 1996;75:432-6.

Shapiro AD, Gilchrist GS, Hoots WK, Cooper H, Gastineau DA. Prospective, randomised trial of two doses of rFVIIa (NovoSeven) in haemophlilia patients with inhibitors undergoing surgery. Thromb Haemost 1998;80:773-8.

Sjamsoedin JM, Leijnen L, Mauser-Bunschoten EP van Geijlswijk JL, van Houwelingen H, van Asten P, Sixma JJ. The effect of activated prothrombon-complex concentrate (FEIBA) on joint and muscle bleeding in patients with hemophilia A and antibodies to factor VIII. N Engl J Med 1981;305:717-21.

Stein SF, Duncan A, Cutler D, Glazer S. (DIC) in a hemophiliac treated with recombinant factor VIIa. Blood 1990;76:438a.

Sumner WT, Monroe DM, Hoffman M. Variability in platelet procoagulant activity in healthy volunteers. Thromb Res 1996;81:533-43.

Wildgoose P, Nemerson Y, Hansen LL, Nielsen FE, Glazer S, Hedner U. Measurement of basal levels of factor VIIa in hemophilia A and B patients. Blood 1992;80:25-8.

8

THE INCIDENCE OF INHIBITORS IN HEMOPHILIA A AND THE INDUCTION OF IMMUNE TOLERANCE

Ernest Briët and Marjolein Peters

Departments of internal medicine and pediatrics

Academic medical center, Amsterdam, The Netherlands

INTRODUCTION

The risk of inhibitor development is highly variable and depends on a number of factors: the definition of risk, the assay method and the threshold level, the persistence of the inhibitor, the frequency of measurements, and also on specific patient factors and treatment factors.

Definition of risk. Risk can be defined as prevalence, incidence rate or cumulative incidence. Prevalence informs us about the percentage of patients in a population with inhibitors at one point in time. It is an important figure if we want to estimate the financial burden caused by inhibitors on a particular center or in a particular state. The incidence rate is the number of new inhibitors divided by the number of patient years. It can be used to compare different products or treatment centers with respect to the frequency of inhibitor development and may help to discover risk factors . Prevalence and incidence rates are related algebraically by the equation: P= IR x D, in which "D" is the duration of the presence of the inhibitor. The cumulative incidence is the percentage of patients who have developed an inhibitor after a certain duration of follow up. It is an interesting figure if we want to explain to an individual patient the risk he is running to get an inhibitor after the

Hemophilia Care in the New Millennium, edited by D. Monroe *et al.*
Kluwer Academic/Plenum Publishers, 2001

exposure to clotting factor concentrates. Cumulative incidence and incidence rates are also related algebraically in the following way: $CI = 1 - e^{-\Sigma(IRxt)}$, in which "t" is the duration of the follow up.

Inhibitor assay. The current inhibitor assay procedure advocated by the Scientific and Standardization Committee of the International Society for Hemostasis and Thrombosis is the Nijmegen modification [1,2] of the Bethesda assay [3]. This modification has increased the specificity of the original assay particularly in the low titer range. Whether we see many inhibitors or few depends also on the exclusion of low titer and transient inhibitors. Low titer inhibitors disappear more frequently than high titer inhibitors. The clinical relevance of this is that it is often possible to continue regular replacement therapy with factor VIII if titers are below five Bethesda Units (BU), while alternative treatments like FEIBA or activated factor VII are usually required if titers are higher.

VARIATION IN THE INCIDENCE OF INHIBITORS

The causes for the wide variation in the frequency of inhibitors are not fully understood. Several factors have been studied and these will be discussed in the following paragraphs. In a meta-analysis of eight single center cohort follow up studies we found cumulative incidences ranging from 2 % up to 46% after follow up of 18 years with an average of 20% for the total group of 451 patients [4]. In order to ensure comparability of the 8 studies we restricted the analysis to patients with severe hemophilia A and to high titer inhibitors. To explain the variability, several factors have been studied and these will be discussed in the following paragraphs.

Severity of hemophilia and mutation types. The old clinical experience that severe hemophilia is more often associated by inhibitors than mild hemophilia has been convincingly confirmed by Hay and his colleagues from the UK hemophilia centers (table 1).

Table 1. The incidence rate of inhibitors in severe hemophilia versus mild or moderately severe hemophilia from the UK hemophilia center directors [5]

	New inhibitors	Number registered	Incidence rate per 1000 patient years
Severe hemophilia	41	1939	3.0
Non severe	16	3061	0.7

Note: included are also low titer and transient inhibitors

The explanation for this difference is probably that the immune system in many patients with severe hemophilia does not recognize factor VIII as a normal human protein by lack of any gene product from the factor VIII gene. Surprisingly therefore, it turned out that there are subgroups of patients with severe hemophilia with relatively low inhibitor frequencies (table 2) [6].

Table 2. The relation of mutation type and inhibitor frequency in patients with severe hemophilia [6]

Mutation type	Number	Inhibitor	%
Missense	69	3	4
Deletion < 200 bp	27	2	7
Inversion 22	125	43	34
Deletion > 200 bp	70	25	36
Stop codon	73	28	38
All mutations	364	101	28

Note: percentages are given since data are lacking for the calculation of formal measures of frequency. Included are also low titer and transient inhibitors

Apparently, some gene product is translated and can be noticed by the immune system in spite of missense mutations or small deletions. Since severe hemophilia A is invariably CRM-negative [7] it can be concluded that immuno-assays are either not sensitive enough to detect these factor VIII fragments or that they are not directed against the circulating epitopes or that the fragments do not reach the circulation.

Immune response genes. Immune response genes have been the target of many studies aimed at explaining the variability of the inhibitor incidence rates. Until now there is no strong evidence that differences in immune response genetic make up contribute in any important way to this variability [8,9]. The well known relation between Hla B27 and disease is associated with relative risks of 18 for reactive arthritis, 37 for Reiter's syndrome and 69 for ankylosing spondylitis. In the case of factor VIII inhibitors, Oldenburg et al report a non significant relative risk of 4.0 for Hla B7 and a non-significant 0.1 for Hla DQA1*0103 [9]. We consider differences in the immune responsiveness the most likely explanation why the majority of patients with large deletions, inversions or stop codons does not get inhibitors. Apparently, our current understanding of the system is insufficient to demonstrate why this is so.

Product associated inhibitors. It would be a major breakthrough if we were able to predict whether a particular product is prone to induce inhibitors. Although there is definitive clinical evidence that some products induce inhibitors more often than others, such a predictive test is not available. The first product associated cluster of inhibitors was described by Peerlinck et al [10] and by Rosendaal et al [11]. These publications concerned a Dutch intermediate purity factor VIII concentrate prepared by controlled pore silica adsorption followed by pasteurization (VIII CPS-P). In the Leuven hemophilia center patients were randomized to receive either this product or a high purity concentrate produced by ion exchange chromatography and a solvent detergent virus inactivation step (VIII SD). Five out of 50 patients treated with VIII CPS-P got an inhibitor versus none out of 61 who received the VIII SD product and the incidence rate was 31 per 1000 patient years [10]. In the Dutch experience with the same VIII CPS-P the incidence rate of inhibitors was also much higher than in patients who were treated with other products (Table 3).

Table 3. The incidence rate of inhibitors associated with factor VIII CPS-P in Leuven and in The Netherlands (NL) with three sources for comparison [10-12]

Study group (reference)	Incidence rate per 1000 patient years	CI95%
Leuven CPS-P [10]	31	9 – 71
NL CPS-P [11]	22	11 – 40
NL historical 1 [11]	5	1 – 31
NL historical 2 [11]	4	4 – 9
USA [12]	6	0.5 – 14

A very similar unfortunate experience occurred with the use of a double virus inactivated product. After worries about the transmission of hepatitis A by SD treated products one company decided to introduce double virus inactivation by pasteurization as well as solvent detergent treatment. Seven out of 33 patients treated with this concentrate developed an inhibitor [13]. An important feature of the inhibitors that occurred in these small epidemics is the fact that these patients had been treated successfully with other products for many years (Table 4).

Table 4. Product associated inhibitors occur after many exposures to factor VIII

VIII Study group (reference)	new inhibitors N	After > 200 exposures N
Product associated inhibitors		
Leuven CPS-P [10]	5	5
Leuven SD+P [13]	8	8
NL CPS-P [11]	11	9
Other inhibitors		
NL historical 1 [11]	4	0
NL historical 2 [11]	2	0
USA [12]	24	0

Other characteristics of these product associated inhibitors are their complex kinetics with incomplete neutralization of factor VIII and the non-linear dose-response in the Bethesda assay as well as the atypical bleeding pattern with a predominance of subcutaneous and intra-muscular rather than joint hemorrhages. Finally, many of these inhibitors are transient after switching to another product or readily responsive to immune tolerance induction [13,14].

Switching products. If some products induce more inhibitors one should expect other products to induce less inhibitors. Considering the many variables that play a role in this adverse immune response it is difficult to study this question. Nevertheless, some patient groups that were treated with one type of product exclusively, had exceptionally low inhibitor cumulative incidence rates [10,15,16]. It is intuitively obvious that the risk of inhibitor formation increases with the exposure to a larger number of products, since every product has a finite chance of containing immune reactive neo-antigens. These three studies support the idea that switching products might be a risk factor for the development of inhibitors [17].

Recombinant products. Since recombinant products are bound to replace plasma derived concentrates in the near future, their safety is of the utmost importance. Two publications describe the occurrence of inhibitors in previously untreated patients who received Recombinate® or Kogenate®. In both studies the cumulative incidence of inhibitors is close to 40% after more than 100 exposures [18,19]. This may seem a high risk in comparison with the findings of older data from the studies mentioned earlier [15,16,20]. However, the surveillance was much more intensive and many of the inhibitors had low titers and were transient. Based on current data we feel that that these products carry similar inhibitor risks as the plasma derived products.

Hemovigilance and post marketing surveillance. Product associated inhibitor formation should not be studied in previously untreated patients since the occurrence of inhibitors in them depends to a large extent on patient factors and any excess risk of inhibitors due to neoantigenicity of the product remains hidden. The evaluation of new products with respect to this side effect should be studied in patients who have proven to tolerate factor VIII. Furthermore, the efficacy studies which are performed for the licensing of new products are usually too small to decide whether the product is associated with an excessive risk of inhibitor formation. To obtain this essential information on the safety of our products, the licensing authorities should enforce post marketing surveillance by granting a conditional license for clinical use of all new products.

INDUCTION OF TOLERANCE

After the daring work of Brackmann in Bonn, several regimens for the induction of tolerance have been evaluated (Table 5). The table provides the briefest summary for each of the schedules but for the details one should consult the original papers[21-26]

Table 5. Schedules for the induction of tolerance in patients with inhibitors against factor VIII

Author(reference)	Regimen	Time to remission (Months)
High dose regimens:		
Brackmann 1977 [21]	Factor VIII 200 U/kg/d + APCC followed by factor VIII 300 U/kg/d	14.5
Nilsson 1988 [22]	Immune adsorption, iv IgG, cyclophosphamide and maintain factor VIII > 30 U/dl	1.3
Smith 1999 [23]	Factor VIII 200 → 100 U/kg/d	3.5
Low dose regimens:		
Ewing 1988 [24]	Factor VIII 50 U/kg/d ± prednisone	3.0
Gruppo 1992 [25]	Factor VIII 100 U/kg/week + immune suppression	12.0
Mauser 1995 [26]	Factor VIII Neutralizing dose followed by 50 U/kg/d <u>or</u> Factor VIII 25 U/kg/2 days	9.0

Cost is one of the major considerations in the decision to start immune tolerance induction treatment. For that reason also it is imperative that we find out whether the dose of factor VIII is a critical factor for the time it takes to reach a tolerant state. The data presented in Table 5 leave room for considerable doubt on this point. In contrast, Mauser-Bunschoten et al. argue that the highest inhibitor titer is a better prognostic factor than the dose of factor VIII. In figure 1 this is illustrated by a comparison of the Kaplan Meier survival curve for the 12 patients with the highest maximum titers (>40 BU) and the 12 patients with the lowest maximum titers (<40 BU).

The authors found no predictive effect for the inhibitor titer at the start of immune tolerance treatment nor for the administration of an antibody neutralizing dose of factor VIII. Very young children seemed to reach tolerance earlier than older patients [26].

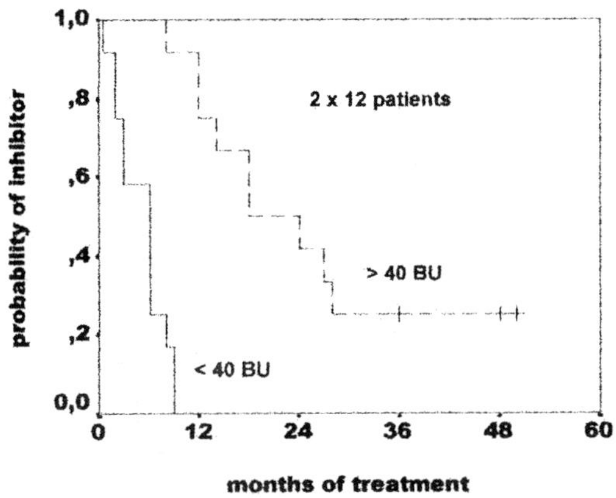

Figure 1. The probability of persistent inhibitor during immune tolerance induction treatment for 12 patients with inhibitor titers > 40 BU versus 12 patients with inhibitor titers < 40 BU. Adapted with permission from Mauser-Bunschoten et al. Blood 1995; 86: 983-988 [26]. Copyright © 1995 American Society of Hematology.

REFERENCES

1. Verbruggen B, Novakova I, Wessels H, Boezeman J, van dB, Mauser-Bunschoten E. The Nijmegen modification of the Bethesda assay for factor VIII:C inhibitors: improved specificity and reliability. Thromb Haemost 1995; 73: 247-251.

2. Giles AR, Verbruggen B, Rivard GE, Teitel J, Walker I. A detailed comparison of the performance of the standard versus the Nijmegen modification of the Bethesda assay in detecting factor VIII:C inhibitors in the haemophilia A population of Canada. Association of Hemophilia Centre Directors of Canada. Factor VIII/IX Subcommittee of Scientific and Standardization Committee of International Society on Thrombosis and Haemostasis. Thromb Haemost 1998; 79: 872-875.

3. Kasper CK, Aledort LM, Counts RB. A more uniformed measurement of factor VIII inhibitors. Thromb Diath Haemorrh 1975; 34: 869-782.

4. Hofmann SL. Southwestern Internal Medicine Conference: Shiga-like toxins in hemolytic-uremic syndrome and thrombotic thrombocytopenic purpura. Am J Med Sci 1993; 306: 398-406.

5. Hay CR, Ludlam CA, Colvin BT, et al. Factor VIII inhibitors in mild and moderate-severity haemophilia A. UK Haemophilia Centre Directors Organisation. Thromb Haemost 1998; 79: 762-766.

6. Schwaab R, Brackmann HH, Meyer C, et al. Haemophilia A: mutation type determines risk of inhibitor formation. Thromb Haemost 1995; 74: 1402-1406.

7. Muller HP, van Tilburg NH, Bertina RM, Veltkamp JJ. Heterogeneity of haemophilia A: a study with three different antisera. Br J Haematol 1982; 52: 485-494.

8. Hay CR, Ollier W, Pepper L, et al. HLA class II profile: a weak determinant of factor VIII inhibitor development in severe haemophilia A. UKHCDO Inhibitor Working Party. Thromb Haemost 1997; 77: 234-237.

9. Oldenburg J, Picard JK, Schwaab R, Brackmann HH, Tuddenham EG, Simpson E. HLA genotype of patients with severe haemophilia A due to intron 22 inversion with and without inhibitors of factor VIII. Thromb Haemost 1997; 77: 238-242.

10. Peerlinck K, Arnout J, Gilles JG, Saint-Remy JM, Vermylen J. A higher than expected incidence of factor VIII inhibitors in multitransfused haemophilia A patients treated with an intermediate purity pasteurized factor VIII concentrate [see comments]. Thromb Haemost 1993; 69: 115-118.

11. Rosendaal FR, Nieuwenhuis HK, Van den Berg HM, et al. A sudden increase in factor VIII inhibitor development in multitransfused hemophilia A patients in The Netherlands. Blood 1993; 81: 2180-2186.

12. McMillan CW, Shapiro SS, Whitehurst D, et al. The natural history of factor VIII:C inhibitors in patients with hemophilia A: A national comparative study. II. Observations on the initial development of factor VIII:C inhibitors. Blood 1988; 71: 344-348.

13. Peerlinck K, Arnout J, Di GM, et al. Factor VIII inhibitors in previously treated haemophilia A patients with a double virus-inactivated plasma derived factor VIII concentrate. Thromb Haemost 1997; 77: 80-86.

14. Mauser-Bunschoten EP, Rosendaal FR, Nieuwenhuis HK, Roosendaal G, Briët E, Van den Berg HM. Clinical course of factor VIII inhibitors developed after exposure to a pasteurised Dutch concentrate compared to classic inhibitors in hemophilia A. Thromb Haemost 1994; 71: 703-706.

15. Guerois C, Laurian Y, Rothschild C, et al. Incidence of factor VIII inhibitor development in severe hemophilia A patients treated only with one brand of highly purified plasma-derived concentrate. Thromb Haemost 1995; 73: 215-218.

16. Yee TT, Williams MD, Hill FG, Lee CA, Pasi KJ. Absence of inhibitors in previously untreated patients with severe haemophilia A after exposure to a single intermediate purity factor VIII product. Thromb Haemost 1997; 78: 1027-1029.

17. Vermylen J. How do some haemophiliacs develop inhibitors?. [Review] [29 refs]. Haemophilia 1998; 4: 538-542.

18. Lusher JM, Arkin S, Abildgaard CF, Schwartz RS, and the Kogenate Previously Untreated Patient Group. Recombinant factor VIII for the treatment of previously untreated patients with hemophilia A--Safety, efficacy, and development of inhibitors. N Engl J Med 1993; 328: 453-459.

19. Bray GL, Gomperts ED, Courter S, et al. A multicenter study of recombinant factor VIII (Recombinate): Safety, efficacy, and inhibitor risk in previously untreated patients with hemophilia A. Blood 1994; 83: 2428-2435.

20. Briët E, Rosendaal FR, Kreuz W, et al. High titer inhibitors in severe haemophilia A. A meta-analysis based on eight long-term follow-up studies concerning inhibitors associated with crude or intermediate purity factor VIII products (letter to the editor). Thromb Haemost 1994; 72: 162-164.

21. Brackmann HH, Oldenburg J, Schwaab R. Immune tolerance for the treatment of factor VIII inhibitors--twenty years' 'bonn protocol'. Vox Sang 1996; 70 Suppl 1: 30-35.

22. Nilsson IM, Berntorp E, Zettervall O. Induction of immune tolerance in patients with hemophilia and antibodies to factor VIII by combined treatment with intravenous IgG, cyclophosphamide and factor VIII. N Engl J Med 1988; 318: 947-950.

23. Smith MP, Spence KJ, Waters EL, et al. Immune tolerance therapy for haemophilia A patients with acquired factor VIII alloantibodies: comprehensive analysis of experience at a single institution. Thromb Haemost 1999; 81: 35-38.

24. Ewing NP, Sanders NL, Dietrich SL, Kasper CK. Induction of immune tolerance to factor VIII in hemophiliacs with inhibitors. JAMA 1988; 259: 65-85.

25. Gruppo RA. Immune tolerance induction with once weekly factor VIII infusions in patients with hemophilia A and inhibitors (abstract). Thromb Haemost 1991; 65 (Suppl): 1168-1168.

26. Mauser-Bunschoten EP, Nieuwenhuis HK, Roosendaal G, van den Berg HM. Low-dose immune tolerance induction in hemophilia A patients with inhibitors. Blood 1995; 86: 983-988.

9

MECHANISMS OF B-CELL TOLERANCE

Marc G. Jacquemin, Beatrijs Vanzieleghem
and Jean-Marie R. Saint-Remy
Center for Molecular and Vascular Biology
University of Leuven, Leuven, Belgium
Address for correspondence:
Jean-Marie R Saint-Remy, MD, PhD,
Center for Molecular and Vascular Biology,
Katholieke Universiteit Leuven,
Campus Gasthuisberg, O&N,
Herestraat 49, B-3000 Leuven, Belgium
tel.: +32-16-345791; fax: +32-16-345990;
e- mail: jeanmarie.saint-remy@med.kuleuven.ac.be

B cells are produced by the bone marrow in which they undergo a series of maturation events as well as several cycles of division. The bone marrow is however also a very efficient organ for the selection of B cells which will be sent out to the periphery and for casting the mature peripheral repertoire. Maturation in the bone marrow is underlined by a successive expression of markers, from intracytoplasmic μ chain to light and δ chains. Five to ten division cycles occur between these steps. Surface expression of IgM pins out the immature B cells, which then progressively mature with expression of surface IgD and loss of intracytoplasmic heavy chains.

Hemophilia Care in the New Millennium, edited by D. Monroe *et al.*
Kluwer Academic/Plenum Publishers, 2001

THE BONE MARROW PROVIDES A CONTINUING HIGH OUTPUT OF B CELLS

The capacity of the bone marrow to produce B cells is impressive. In a mouse, it has been estimated that about 10 to 20 x 10^6 B cells are formed every day, which allows a quick extrapolation to the number of B cells produced in man, taken into account that a mouse weighs only 15 to 20 gr. Interestingly enough, the number of mature B cells that actually leave the bone marrow is about a tenth of that produced, showing that efficient selection mechanisms are at play. Further, 7 out of 10 B cells die prematurely in the periphery, leaving about 3% of the initial production, namely 3 to 6 x 10^5, ready to replenish the peripheral B cell pool. This sets the stage for B cells: there is a continuing high turnover of B cells which seemingly lasts as long as the organism lives. T cells, by contrast, which are also produced by the bone marrow but have to be educated in the thymus, constitute a pool which is essentially constituted at birth; the thymus undergoes rapid involution after birth.

B CELLS HAVE A HIGH CAPACITY TO DIVERSIFY

A second hallmark of B cells is a very high potential for diversification. This relies on essentially two mechanisms: immunoglobulin gene rearrangement and somatic hypermutation. The variable region gene coding for the heavy (H) chain is made of three segments, V, J and D. The VH segment is made of 7 or 8 families with a number of members in each of them, varying from 4 to 100. In man, 10 to 20 different D segments have been defined, and 9 different JH segments. During variable gene rearrangement, random association of one V with one D and one J segment occurs. The variable region genes for the κ light chain are made of about 100 V segments and a few J segments, while about 30 members have been described within the Vλ family. Randomly associated heavy chain V, D and J segments combine in random order with randomly associated either V and J segments of the κ chain or V segments of the λ chain, providing therefore an almost infinite number of possible V chain combinations. This mainly occurs in the bone marrow.

The second mechanism, i.e. somatic hypermutation, is an antigen-driven phenomenon which occurs in the germinal centers of secondary follicles during the mounting of secondary (or subsequent) immune responses. Hypermutation of variable regions occurs under the influence of T cells and results in amino acid substitution primarily at the level of hypervariable regions. Each variable chain contains three hypervariable regions named CDR1 to 3 for 'complementarity-determining region'. These CDRs form the actual region of antibody coming in close contact with antigen epitopes. The 6 CDRs, 3 on the variable region of both the light and the heavy chains, constitute the antibody paratope or antigen-binding region. Mutations introduced in CDRs provide therefore another degree of diversity for mature antibody molecules.

The peripheral pool of B cells is shaped by a combination of deletion and anergy. (1) The high output of B cells from the bone marrow and the extraordinary potential for diversification resulting from random gene rearrangement is accompanied by an increased likelihood of generating self-reactive B cell clones. In fact a combination of deletion and anergy-inducing mechanisms shape the B cell repertoire in an efficient manner. The clonal selection hypothesis, which was formulated more than 30 years ago, was based on the assumption that B cells are unipotential, a postulate which has resisted intensive investigation. It was thought that B cells encountering self antigens were deleted while other B cells underwent a series of maturational steps towards a functional state. However, it is now clear that whenever a B cell meets a self antigen, the outcome is not necessarily deletion. Such an encountering can indeed result in cell maturation or induction of tolerance, as will be discussed below.

B cell deletion occurs in the bone marrow, a process which is seemingly efficient if one considers that only 10% of the produced B cells actually leave the bone marrow. However, it is now well established that a significant proportion of self-reactive B cells do escape deletion and accumulate in the T-cell zones of the spleen where they die rapidly. The precise significance of this second site for deletion is not entirely clear, but this phenomenon may account for the transitory presence of self-reactive B cells in the periphery.

CROSS-LINKING OF SURFACE IG AND AFFINITY THRESHOLD DETERMINE THE FATE OF B CELLS

Tolerance occurs through cross-linking of surface Ig and this requires a minimum threshold affinity. Cross-linking is easily achieved with multivalent antigens and indeed tolerance is readily induced to surface self antigens. However, monovalent antigens do not induce tolerance, which allows the passage of self reactive B cells in the periphery. The second condition to be fulfilled is a minimum threshold affinity. High-affinity interaction leads to deletion, but intermediate affinity results in anergy. Low affinity interaction results in anergy for surface self antigen, but ignorance for soluble self antigens. The end result of this double selection mechanism is that the peripheral B cell population pool is heterogeneous, including self-reactive cells to monovalent antigens and low affinity B cells to soluble antigens, together with a mixed population of anergized B cells (Figures 1 and 2).

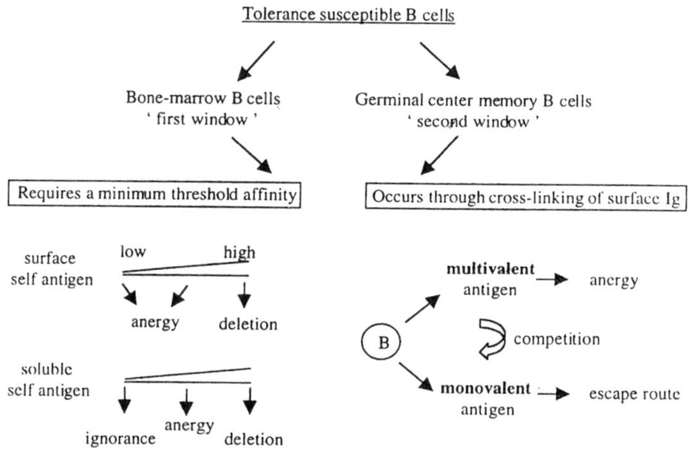

Figure 1

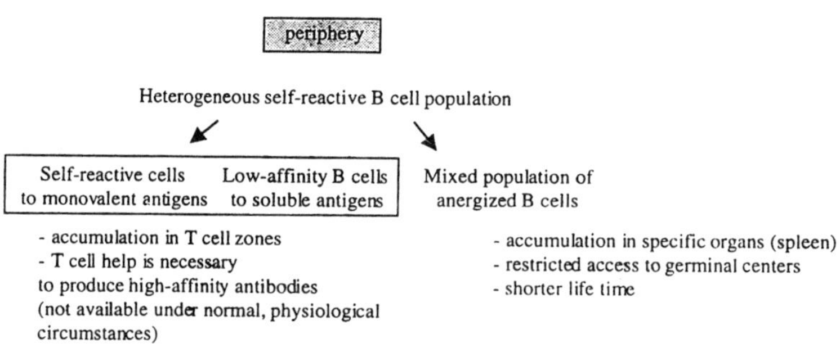

Figure 2

B CELL ANERGY INDUCTION IS AN ACTIVE PROCESS

Tolerance induction at the B cell level has two main characteristics. First, it is the result of an active signaling process generated at the surface of B cells. Second, it is a reversible phenomenon, at least to some extent. Whether the B cell maturational stage rather than to the age of the animal itself is a key factor in tolerance susceptibility, or whether B cells can be anergized at any stage is not yet decided. For the sake of clarity, one can distinguish three stages at which B cells are particularly amenable to anergy induction. Mouse neo-natal B cells are a classical example of tolerance susceptibility, corresponding to the first 4 or 5 days immediately after birth. However, this can not be merely extrapolated to humans: a human fetus is able to mount an immune response as soon as the fourth gestation month. The other two stages at which tolerance can be induced are the bone marrow B cells just after first expansion, what is usually called the 'first window' of tolerance susceptibility. Very importantly, however, a 'second window' exists, which corresponds to the stage at which B memory cells are generated.

Most of current knowledge about tolerance has been gained through the use of transgenic animals, which produce a significant proportion of B cells expressing identical antigen receptors to either a self antigen or to an antigen injected at high doses. The fate of B cells can therefore be easily followed by detection of surface markers. Some caution should however be exerted when interpreting the results obtained in such animals. Transgenic mice have an accelerated development of B cells as compared to the physiological situation and some of the maturation steps appear to be truncated. Besides, there is no competition by the normal B cell repertoire in such model systems.

B CELL ANERGY IS REVERSIBLE

This is of importance as anergy can be reversed. Removal of the tolerogen during the initial phase of tolerance induction can restore normal responsiveness. In addition, three main situations can lead to reverse anergy: extensive cross-linking of surface Ig, which can compensate for relatively low affinity, help provided by T cells, or triggering signals supplied by cytokines such as IL-4. These last two circumstances at least could have a clinical counterpart when tissue destruction, infection or inflammation bring about unusual T cell activation and a burst of pro-inflammatory cytokines. (See figure 3, next page.)

B cell tolerance is reversible:

- when the tolerogen is removed (lag period)

- by extensive receptor cross-linking which compensates for relatively low affinity (final deletion?)

- through help provided by T cells during
  tissue destruction
  infection
  inflammation

- by triggering signals provided by cytokines (i.e., IL-4) or anti-CD40 antibodies

B CELL ANERGY CAN STILL BE INDUCED DURING SECONDARY IMMUNE RESPONSES

The generation of B memory cells is accompanied by somatic hypermutation. The introduction of mutations in the antigen-combining sites of antibodies is a necessary step for increasing antibody affinity during the maturation of immune responses. However, it also carries the risk of generating novel anti-self specificities. Fortunately, B cells are still susceptible to be anergized or deleted at this stage by mechanisms similar to those occurring in the bone marrow.

B CELL ANERGY AND DELETION ARE NOT NECESSARILY DISTINCT PHENOMENA

An important issue concerns the fate of anergized B cells. It seems well established that such B cells have a shorter lifespan than mature B cells, which interestingly blurs the distinction between anergy and deletion. Anergized B cells accumulate in specific regions of the spleen or lymphoid organs and have restricted access to germinal centers. However, an additional phenomenon, which has been observed more recently and is of direct relevance to the mechanisms of B cell anergy induction, is the demonstration that B cells can be killed by T cells. Cells express surface receptors which, after activation, transduce signals leading to apoptosis. One of such receptors is Fas: increased expression of Fas at the surface of B cells is obtained by activation through the CD40 antigen, or possibly through intense and/or prolonged stimulation via the Ig receptor. B cells expressing Fas are targets for Th1 cells expressing the corresponding Fas ligand. Interestingly this effect is counteracted by binding of IL-4 to its specific receptor also expressed at B cell surface.

B CELL AUTO-REACTIVITY IS KEPT UNDER CONTROL

From all the above-described events, it can be concluded that mature B cells reacting with self antigens are present in the periphery, either because they have not had any contact with self antigen or because such a contact did not lead to cell deletion. Does this mean that auto-immune reactivity is an ineluctable consequence? Fortunately a number of safeguards exist, some of which have already been alluded to above. B cells reacting to self membrane antigens are easily eliminated or anergized. Self-reactive B cells in the periphery do interact with antigen with only low affinity. In addition, the "second window" of anergy susceptibility during the generation of B memory cells offers an additional opportunity to eliminate clones that have acquired higher affinity to self antigens. It should also be stressed that without T cell help, B cells have no capacity to produce high-affinity antibodies: such T cell help is not available in the periphery under normal, physiological conditions.

The concept of idiotypic regulation finds here its logical place. An idiotype collectively refers to the ensemble of determinants (idiotopes) carried by an antigen receptor at the level of its variable part. This involves soluble antibody molecules and surface Ig expressed by B cells, but also the variable part of the antigen receptor of T cells. The importance of network interactions between corresponding idiotypes for the regulation of immune responses in general, and in the maintenance of tolerance in particular, has been the matter of numerous pro and con debates. Overwhelming evidence in favor of a significant role for idiotypic interactions has however been provided, which can be easily integrated within the context of B cell anergy. Thus, both animals and men spontaneously produce anti-idiotypic antibodies together with antibodies elicited to the immunizing agent. That such anti-idiotypic antibodies modulate the initial response is well established. Anti-idiotypic antibodies specific to self-reactive antibodies play a role in homeostasis of the anti self response and as such could be considered as representing a third level at which tolerance is maintained.

Anti-idiotypic antibodies can neutralize an effector, such as a specific antibody to factor VIII. However, they can modulate the function of B or T cells expressing the corresponding idiotype. Interestingly, in studies carried out with human lymphoma, it was shown that anti-idiotypic antibodies could also induce target cell apoptosis, which adds another dimension to the potential interest of such antibodies in B cell anergy mechanisms. Whether this effect can occur spontaneously or only as the result of hyperimmunization with an idiotype is not known.

B CELLS REACTIVE TO FACTOR VIII ARE PRESENT IN THE PERIPHERY

Observations made in healthy donors have demonstrated that anti-factor VIII antibodies were indeed present in the normal repertoire (2).

This not only confirmed previous observations on the presence of auto-antibodies to major self proteins, but added a new functional dimension. Indeed, after affinity purification, anti-factor VIII antibodies from healthy donors exhibited the capacity to inhibit the function of factor VIII as efficiently as antibodies produced by hemophilia patients on substitutive therapy (3). The reason why no inhibition of factor VIII activity is detectable in serum was at least in part due to the presence of corresponding anti-idiotypic antibodies.

In mild/moderate hemophilia A patients an increased frequency of inhibitor has been observed associated with mutations occurring in a ± 100 amino acid-long sequence located at the junction of the C1 and C2 domains (4). Mild hemophilia is of particular interest for the study of tolerance to factor VIII. In such case, the level of circulating factor VIII antigen is close to normal, which should have allowed patients to become tolerant towards factor VIII, except for the determinants that are directly or indirectly dependent of the mutation site. It is therefore to be expected that the number of epitopes primarily recognized by antibodies (as well as T cells) would be limited. Recent evidence obtained from the analysis of a patient with a mutation in the carboxy-terminal end of the C1 domain has shown that the point substitution had destroyed a B cell epitope normally present on wild-type factor VIII, as antibodies (both polyclonal and monoclonal) prepared from this patient bound to and inhibited only wild-type factor VIII (5). This B cell epitope appears therefore important for tolerance induction.

B CELL TOLERANCE AND THERAPY OF INHIBITORS

Infusion of high doses of factor VIII for the treatment of inhibitor patients can result in disappearance of detectable plasma inhibitors, the exact mechanism of which is not elucidated. On theoretical grounds the levels of circulating factor VIII obtained by such treatment is sufficient to cross-link surface Ig and induce anergy at the B cell level (or T cell level, although with lower antigen concentrations). This awaits formal investigation. However, a mechanism that is likely to play a role here is the induction of anti-idiotypic antibodies, as we recently demonstrated for two hemophilia patients under factor VIII infusion therapy (6). The success or failure of infusion of high doses of factor VIII is likely to be related to the underlying condition: bleeding, inflammation or infection all lead to higher level of T cell activation which then provides B cells with sufficient help as to break the state of tolerance.

On the other hand, an increasing number of possible novel strategies for therapy of factor VIII inhibitors are identified from the accumulating knowledge of the mechanisms of anergy induction. Interfering between B and T cells with molecules that inhibit secondary signals is a promising approach. This can be achieved by using antibodies directed towards surface receptors such as CD40 ligand (7), B7 molecules, or soluble protein such as CTLA-4. Tolerance can indeed be obtained at the T cell level with such reagents. Another possible avenue is to design methods by which it becomes feasible to actively induce a production of anti-idiotypic antibodies specific to anti-factor VIII antibodies, a mechanism by which a physiological state of factor VIII unresponsiveness could be re-established.

From the above discussion it should appear that the mechanisms responsible for anergy induction at the B cell level result in an intricate network of interactions between B and T cell on the one hand, and self protein on the other hand. The population of B cells found in the periphery is heterogeneous not only in terms of specificity and affinity for antigen recognition, but also with regard to its state of responsiveness to self proteins, including lifespan and re-circulating properties. This however offers a number of possibilities for intervention which will no doubt be the matter of extensive studies in the forthcoming years.

REFERENCES

The interested reader is referred to key references such as:

1. Klinman NR (1996) The "clonal selection hypothesis" and current concepts of B cell tolerance, *Immunity* 5: 189-95; Nossal GJV (1994) Negative selection of lymphocytes, *Cell* **76**: 229-239; Pulendran B, Kannourakis G, Nouri S, Smith KGC, and Nossal GJV (1995) Soluble antigen can cause enhanced apoptosis of grminal centre B cells Nature **375**: 331-334; Shokat KM, and Goodnow CC (1995) Antigen-induced B-cell death and elimination during germinal-centre immune responses Nature **375**: 334-338; Fulcher DA, and Basten A (1997) B-cell activation versus tolerance – The central role of immunoglobulin receptor engagement and T-cell help. Intern. Rev. Immunol. **15**: 33-52; Liu YJ (1997) Sites of B lymphocyte selection, activation, and tolerance in spleen. J exp Med **186**: 625-629; Rajewsky K (1996) Clonal selection and learning in the antibody system Nature **381**: 751-758; Coutinho A, Kazatchkine MD, and Avrameas S (1995) Natural autoantibodies, *Curr Opin Immunol* **7**: 812-818; Cook MC, Basten A, and Fazekas de St. Groth B (1997) Outer periarteriolar lymphoid sheath arrest and subsequent differentiation of both naive and tolerant immunoglobulin transgenic B cells is determined by B cell receptor occupancy, *J Exp Med* **186**: 631-43; Adelstein S, Pritchard-Briscoe H, Anderson TA, Crosbie J, Gammon G, Loblay RH, Basten A, and Goodnow CC (1991) Induction of self-tolerance in T cells but not B cells of transgenic mice expressing little self antigen, *Science* **251**: 1223-1225; Johnson JG, and Jemmerson R (1992) Tolerance induction in resting memory B cells specific for a protein antigen, *J Immunol* **148**: 2682-2689; Shokat KM, and Goodnow CC (1995) Antigen-induced B-cell death and elimination during germinal-centre immune responses, *Nature* **375**: 334-338.

2. Sultan, Y., M. Kazatchkine, P. Maisonneuve, and U. Nydegger (1984) Anti-idiotypic suppression of auto-antibodies to factor VIII (anti-hemophilic factor) by high dose intravenous gammaglobulin. *Lancet.* 2:765-766.

3. Gilles JGG, and Saint-Remy JMR (1994) Healthy subjects produce both anti-factor VIII and specific anti-idiotypic antibodies J Clin Invest. **94**: 1496-1505

4. Hay CR, Ludlam CA, Colvin BT, Hill FG, Preston FE, Wasseem N, Bagnall R, Peake IR, on behalf of the UK Haemophilia Centre Directors Organisaton, and: Berntop E, Mauser-Bunschoten EP, Fijnvandraat K, Kasper K, White G, and Santagostino E (1998) Factor VIII inhibitors in Mild and Moderate-severity Haemophilia A Thromb. Haemost. **79**:762-766

5. Jacquemin MG, Benhida A, Peerlinck K, Desqueper BG, Vander Elst L, Lavend'homme R, d'Oiron R, Schwaab R, Bakkus M, Thielemans K, Gilles JGG, Vermylen J, and Saint-Remy JMR (1999) A human antibody directed to the factor VIII C1 domain inhibits factor VIII cofactor activity and binding to von Willebrand factor ***manuscript in revision (Blood)***

6. Gilles JG, Desqueper B, Lenk H, Vermylen J, and Saint-Remy JMR (1996) Neutralising anti-idiotypic antibodies to factor VIII inhibitors following desensitization in patients with hemophilia A. J. Clin. Invest. **97**: 1382-1388

7. Foy TM, Aruffo A, Bajorath J, Buhlmann JE, and Noelle RJ (1996) Immune regulation by CD40 and its ligand GP39 (1996) Annu. Rev. Immunol. **14**: 591-617

10
MECHANISMS OF UNRESPONSIVENESS: T- AND B-CELL MEDIATED MECHANISMS OF ANERGY

Roberta Greenwood and Jeffrey Frelinger
Department of Microbiology and Immunology
University of North Carolina – Chapel Hill
Chapel Hill, NC 27599

Introduction

In this chapter we will attempt to briefly review the relevant immunological concepts concerning both T and B cell unresponsiveness. We will focus on the broad concepts, and use them to frame the problems of gene therapy related to hemophilia.

Since the seminal paper of Owen in 1945, it has been appreciated that the lack of immune responses to self proteins is an acquired rather than an innate process (1). By the nature of the generation of diversity, receptors for both T and B cells are produced that are able to bind to self proteins. The mechanisms by which these cells are controlled are only now being understood. It is important to note that the maturation processes for T cells not only allow but require that they have a measurable affinity for self proteins and this may also be true for B cells, thus setting the stage for autoreactivity.

T CELL DEVELOPMENT

T cell precursors are produced in the bone marrow and migrate to the thymus for their development. The different stages of T cell development are distinguished based on the surface expression of the co-receptors CD4 and CD8 [See (2) for

Hemophilia Care in the New Millennium, edited by D. Monroe *et al.*
Kluwer Academic/Plenum Publishers, 2001

review]. Newly arrived T cells in the thymus lack expression of CD4 and CD8 and the T cell receptor (TCR). These double negative ($CD4^-/CD8^-$) cells proliferate and differentiate in the thymus. They rearrange their TCR α and β genes to connect variable, joining, and constant regions (and diversity for β) to produce a very diverse array of TCRs that recognize a wide range of antigens. The cells express their TCRs and both CD4 and CD8. After the TCRs are expressed at the cell surface, the cells are selected based on the binding capabilities of their TCRs. The TCRs are tested for binding to the major histocompatibility complex (MHC) molecules present in the thymus. The MHC molecules in the thymus that the T cells are selected against contain peptides from many different self proteins. The T cells that bind with high affinity to the MHC-self peptide complex die (negative selection) (3). Those T cells that express TCRs with low affinity for the MHC-peptide complexes survive, while those that do not bind also die. This process is called positive selection (4). Between positive and negative selection more than 90% of the original double positive T cells die. As a result of engagement of either the CD4 or CD8 co-receptor by MHC class II or class I complexes T cells stop producing the other co-receptor, resulting in single positive cells that express only CD4 or CD8. These naive CD4 or CD8 T cells are released into the peripheral immune system where they can encounter antigen.

Not all of the self-reactive T cells are eliminated by negative selection. Some self proteins have tissue specific expression or are developmentally regulated such that they are not present in the thymus during T cell selection. T cells that recognize peptides from these proteins are not eliminated in the thymus and reach the periphery. It is evident from the process of selection in the thymus that a degree of self reactivity is necessary for T cells to survive selection because the T cells must express a TCR that binds with low affinity to a MHC-self peptide complex. Therefore, the production of self-reactive T cells is inherent in the way in which T cells develop.

Peripheral Unresponsiveness

T Cell Anergy

Clearly, T cell activation must be carefully regulated. Activation of a naive T cell requires two signals. The first signal is provided by the TCR binding to the MHC-peptide complex. The second signal can be provided by the binding of CD80 (B7.1) or CD86 (B7.2) on the antigen presenting cell (APC) to CD28 on the T cell. Together these two signals result in the synthesis of new proteins such as activation markers, cytokines, interleukin-2 (IL-2) receptors, etc. This stimulates proliferation and differentiation of T cells. In the absence of the second signal T cells enter a state of anergy. Anergy is a state of unresponsiveness in which the T cell is refractory to stimulation. This state can be reversed by exposure to IL-2 (5) or removal of the stimulus.

Many self-reactive peripheral T cells are maintained in an unresponsive or anergic state through the absence of costimulation. Depending on the type of cell that displays the MHC-peptide complex to the T cell, costimulation may or may not be provided. Some cells such as activated B cells, mature dendritic cells, and macrophage express high levels of CD80 and CD86. These cells provide costimulation and are often referred to as professional APC. Most other cells lack high levels of CD80 and CD86. Antigen presentation by these cells fails to stimulate T cells and results in a state of anergy.

T Cell Ignorance

The concentration of some self proteins is low enough that T cells that recognize them never effectively encounter the antigen. This is referred to as T cell ignorance and it prevents self recognition of proteins that are present in low concentrations. Other self proteins are sequestered in privileged sites that exclude T cells. Again, through T cell ignorance a response to self protein is prevented. Examples of T cell ignorance are myelin basic protein in the central nervous system, and peptide hormones that are present in very low concentrations.

B CELL DEVELOPMENT

B cell precursors are produced and develop in the bone marrow. The different stages in B cell development are distinguished by the gene rearrangements and surface expression of the immunoglobulin heavy and light chains [See (6) for review]. In the pro-B cell stage the immunoglobulin heavy chain genes rearrange. If rearrangement of a heavy chain gene is productive, the heavy chain is expressed at the cell surface with a surrogate light chain. Cells that express a heavy chain at the cell surface proliferate. During the pre-B cell stage the κ and/or λ light chain genes rearrange. If a functional light chain is formed, it replaces the surrogate light chains and IgM is expressed at the cell surface, producing an immature B cell. The surface IgM on immature B cells is tested for binding to self proteins. If the IgM receptors bind self protein with high affinity, the B cell dies. This removes many, but not all of the self-recognizing B cells. For some B cells there is a second chance to produce a functional IgM antibody that does not recognize self. Some self-recognizing immature B cells that bind to self antigen will rearrange another light chain in a process called receptor editing. Immature B cells exit the bone marrow to continue their differentiation in the spleen. The B cells that survive selection begin to express IgD as well as IgM. These are mature B cells that circulate in the peripheral immune system.

There is a great decrease in cell number between the bone marrow and the B cells that reach the periphery. Only 10-20% of the immature B cells become part of the peripheral B cell population. B cells may be positively selected for expressing immunoglobulin with low affinity binding to self proteins in the bone marrow. Positive selection may also take place in the peripheral immune system where binding weakly to self or foreign antigens may be required for long term survival of B cells. Thus, it is possible that self recognition is a requirement in the maturation processes of B cells as well as T cells.

Like the selection of T cells in the thymus, the process of negative selection of B cells is not complete in the bone marrow and many self-recognizing B cells are released into the peripheral immune system. Self-recognizing antibodies that bind to self proteins such as collagen, myoglobin and transferrin can be isolated (7). These self-recognizing B cells are controlled in a number of different ways.

Much of what is known about the regulation of self-recognizing B cells has come from studies in transgenic mouse model systems. In one model immunoglobulin transgenic mice were produced in which most B cells make antibodies that recognize hen egg lysozyme (HEL) (8). These mice were crossed with transgenic mice that produce a soluble form of HEL as a self protein. In the doubly transgenic offspring the T and B cell responses to different levels of HEL expression could be studied. At high concentrations of HEL there was a drastic reduction in the number of cells producing antibody that recognized HEL and the antibodies produced by the remaining cells had decreased affinities for HEL. Thus, at high concentrations of self antigen the B cells that recognize the antigen are eliminated.

At very low concentrations of HEL (10^{-10}M) B cells were present that produced antibodies that had high affinities for HEL. This indicates that a threshold concentration of self protein is required for the elimination of self-recognizing B cells.

Hemophilia

B cells

Normal treatment for hemophilia is the infusion of the missing or nonfunctional clotting factor to control or prevent bleeding episodes. Factor VIII is given to hemophilia A patients and factor IX is given to hemophilia B patients. A serious complication in these treatments is the development of inhibitors. Inhibitors are antibodies against factor VIII or factor IX that develop in an individual after treatment. They develop in approximately 20% of hemophilia A patients and approximately 5% of hemophilia B patients. Inhibitors bind to factor VIII or factor IX, preventing function. In some patients with inhibitors the injection of factor VIII or factor IX causes an anamnestic response. Thus, inhibitor development makes the normal treatment for hemophilia become ineffective or even dangerous. In these cases other treatments must be used to control bleeding.

As previously mentioned healthy individuals have antibodies to many different self proteins. Antibodies that recognize factor VIII can often be found in healthy individuals. In one study anti-factor VIII antibodies were detected in the whole plasma of 85 out of 500 (17%) of nonhemophilic individuals (9). In a separate study, using immunoadsorption techniques, Gilles et al. detected anti-factor VIII antibodies in 10 out of 10 normal donors (10). Some of these antibodies even had an inhibitory effect on factor VIII function. Acquired factor VIII inhibitors occur in about .2-1 individuals per million.

Anti-factor IX antibodies have not been reported in healthy individuals, though very rare cases of acquired inhibitors do occur. The differences in size and serum concentrations may explain why factor VIII is more immunogenic than factor IX. The amino acid sequence of factor VIII is over 5 times longer than that of factor IX. The greater length of factor VIII provides many more potential antibody binding sites as well as T cell epitopes. The molar concentration of factor VIII is about 270 times lower than the concentration of factor IX. Factor VIII is normally present at about 100 ng/ml, while factor IX is normally present at about 5 μg/ml. The low concentration of factor VIII is nearer the threshold required for the elimination of self-recognizing B cells, which might allow some factor VIII recognizing B cells to escape deletion.

T cells

There is good evidence that T cells participate in the formation of inhibitors to factor VIII by providing T cell help. In one study Singer et al. demonstrated that T cells from inhibitor patients proliferate in response to factor VIII (11). This suggests that inhibitor patients have factor VIII recognizing T cells that are capable of responding to antigen. More evidence is provided by three studies that demonstrated that as some HIV^{+} hemophilia patients lose $CD4^{+}$ T cells, they also lose inhibitors to factor VIII (12-14). Thus, as $CD4^{+}$ T cells are lost, B cells can no longer produce antibodies to factor VIII. This suggests that factor VIII recognizing T cells are required for the immune response to factor VIII.

In the study by Singer et al. T cells from some of the inhibitor negative individuals and some of the normal control individuals had a proliferative response to factor VIII, though the responses were lower than those from inhibitor patients (11). It is possible that T cells that recognize FVIII often escape deletion in the thymus and are common in healthy individuals.

T cell responses to factor IX have not been reported in inhibitor patients or in healthy individuals. It is possible that immune responses to factor IX are less frequent than those to factor VIII because of the differences in size and concentration of these two clotting factors as described above.

GENE THERAPY

There is hope that in the future hemophilia can be treated by gene therapy. The advantages of gene therapy over current treatments are a continuous supply of clotting factor, no possibility of contamination, and avoiding the high cost of purifying clotting factor. Hemophilia A and B are ideal candidates for treatment with gene therapy for a number of reasons. They are both single gene disorders. Functional clotting factor can be produced by a variety of cell types. A low level of expression (1-10% of normal) can have a significant clinical effect, and expression does not need to be tightly regulated.

A barrier to long term gene expression following gene transfer is the immune response to the newly expressed factor VIII or factor IX. The presence of inhibitors in some hemophilia patients demonstrates that both factor VIII and factor IX can be immunogenic. T cells and B cells recognizing factor VIII may be quite common given that normal individuals have factor VIII recognizing antibodies and T cells that respond to factor VIII.

Factor VIII

Studies transferring human factor VIII into normal mice, hemophilia mice, and hemophilia dogs have shown some encouraging success for long term expression, although there is evidence for immune responses to the transferred factor VIII. In one study intravenous administration of adenovirus encoding human factor VIII (B domain deleted) resulted in long term (22 weeks) expression of low levels (40 ng/ml) of factor VIII in normal mice (15). The authors did not detect any factor VIII antibodies by western analysis. In a separate study factor VIII was transferred into two strains of factor VIII knockout mice. This transfer initially produced high expression of factor VIII in the plasma (over 2000 mU/ml--normal is 1000 mU/ml), but with time this expression decreased to 20-200 mU/ml (16). By ELISA analysis, the authors detected low levels of factor VIII recognizing antibodies in some of the mice that may have contributed to the decrease in expression. In the dog model for hemophilia this same transfer technique resulted in the development of antibodies against human factor VIII (17). The expression of the factor VIII was limited to 7-10 days possibly because of the antibodies against factor VIII.

Factor IX

A number of different viral vectors and transfer techniques have been employed to introduce factor IX into mice. Many of these studies have demonstrated the production of antibodies against factor IX. In the context of gene therapy these antibodies could inhibit factor IX function as well as reduce its half-life in the blood and prevent further treatments with exogenous factor IX.

Some of these studies demonstrated that factor IX expression could be extended by suppressing the immune response. Dai et al. used adenovirus to transfer canine factor IX into nude mice (T cell deficient) where expression lasted for a year (18). When they repeated this transfer in normal mice, the levels of factor IX decreased rapidly. This decrease occurred in both μMT/μMT mice, which lack B cells and β_2-microglobulin knockout mice (deficient in class I expression), indicating that both antibody and cytotoxic T cells contribute to the decline in expression. The authors were able to extend expression in normal mice by treating with the immunosuppressive drugs cyclophosphamide and cyclosporine A.

In a separate study Poller et al. demonstrated that the immunosuppressive effects that the E3 region of adenovirus exerts on class I expression could extend the time that human factor IX is expressed in mice (19). They also discovered that depleting CD4+ cells with antibody injections could increase this time period. Stein et al. immunosuppressed mice by depleting macrophage with clodronate liposomes and inhibited T and B cell interactions by treatments with antibodies to CD40 ligand (20). This prolonged expression of human factor IX from an adenovirus infection. The treatment reduced antibodies to adenovirus and decreased IL-10 and IFN-γ levels.

The immune response stimulated by adeno-associated virus (AAV) infection is reduced compared to adenovirus. This may also decrease the immune response to factor IX by reducing bystander activation. Using AAV to transfer factor IX into mice has resulted in long term expression in some studies (21-24). However, antibodies against factor IX were detected even with AAV gene transfer (22, 23, 25). The expression of factor IX from AAV is extended in the absence of an immune response much like adenoviral driven expression. Herzog et al. transferred human factor IX into Rag-1 knockout mice, which lack functional B and T cells (25). They demonstrated long term expression of factor IX in this system.

Even in the absence of any viral vector, human factor IX can be immunogenic in mice. Using naked DNA injections Katsumi and his colleagues demonstrated both antibodies and CTL directed against human factor IX in mice (26).

Besides studying gene therapy in mice some researchers have also examined factor IX expression in dogs. Snyder et al. used AAV to transfer canine factor IX into dogs that lack functional factor IX (23). They observed long term expression of very low levels of factor IX. The authors did not find inhibiting antibodies in the 2 dogs they studied, using the Bethesda assay. In a second study by Herzog et al. in which canine factor IX was transferred with AAV into dogs lacking functional factor IX, two of the five dogs developed antibodies to factor IX with one of the two having inhibiting antibodies (27). This demonstrates that the immune response to gene therapy can be a problem in the large animal model for hemophilia B as it is in mice.

Conclusions

In the normal treatment of hemophilia patients it is important to avoid stimulating T and B cell responses that lead to inhibitors. In any future treatments of hemophilia by gene therapy it will be important to avoid stimulating these T and B cell responses and also potential cytotoxic T cell responses. Currently little is known about what stimulates some patients to develop inhibitors, while other patients do not. A better understanding of the how the immune responses to factor VIII and IX are initiated and regulated would help in avoiding the generation of inhibitors and make treatment of hemophilia by gene therapy more feasible. It should be possible to render T cells unresponsive to factor VIII or factor IX by inducing anergy.

References

1. **Owen, R.** 1945. Immunogenetic consequences of vascular anastamoses between bovine twins. *Science 102:400.*
2. **Res, P., and H. Spits.** 1999. Developmental stages in the human thymus. *Seminars in Immunology 11:39.*
3. **Nossal, G. J.** 1994. Negative selection of lymphocytes. *Cell 76:229.*
4. **von Boehmer, H.** 1994. Positive selection of lymphocytes. *Cell 76:219.*
5. **Beverly, B., S. M. Kang, M. J. Lenardo, and R. H. Schwartz.** 1992. Reversal of in vitro T cell clonal anergy by IL-2 stimulation. *Int Immunol 4:661.*

6. **Benschop, R. J., and J. C. Cambier.** 1999. B cell development: signal transduction by antigen receptors and their surrogates. *Curr Opin Immunol 11:143.*

7. **Guilbert, B., G. Dighiero, and S. Avrameas.** 1982. Naturally occurring antibodies against nine common antigens in human sera. I. Detection, isolation and characterization. *J Immunol 128:2779.*

8. **Goodnow, C. C.** 1992. Transgenic mice and analysis of B-cell tolerance. *Annu Rev Immunol 10:489.*

9. **Algiman, M., G. Dietrich, U. E. Nydegger, D. Boieldieu, Y. Sultan, and M. D. Kazatchkine.** 1992. Natural antibodies to factor VIII (anti-hemophilic factor) in healthy individuals. *Proc Natl Acad Sci U S A 89:3795.*

10. **Gilles, J. G., and J. M. Saint-Remy.** 1994. Healthy subjects produce both anti-factor VIII and specific anti- idiotypic antibodies. *J Clin Invest 94:1496.*

11. **Singer, S. T., J. E. Addiego, Jr., D. C. Reason, and A. H. Lucas.** 1996. T lymphocyte proliferative responses induced by recombinant factor VIII in hemophilia A patients with inhibitors. *Thromb Haemost 76:17.*

12. **Leyva, W. H., A. P. Knutsen, and J. H. Joist.** 1988. Disappearance of a high response factor VIII inhibitor in a hemophiliac with AIDS. *Am J Clin Pathol 89:414.*

13. **Bray, G. L., B. L. Kroner, S. Arkin, L. W. Aledort, M. W. Hilgartner, M. E. Eyster, M. V. Ragni, and J. J. Goedert.** 1993. Loss of high-responder inhibitors in patients with severe hemophilia A and human immunodeficiency virus type 1 infection: a report from the Multi-Center Hemophilia Cohort Study. *Am J Hematol 42:375.*

14. **Ragni, M. V., F. A. Bontempo, and J. H. Lewis.** 1989. Disappearance of inhibitor to factor VIII in HIV-infected hemophiliacs with progression to AIDS or severe ARC. *Transfusion 29:447.*

15. **Connelly, S., J. M. Gardner, R. M. Lyons, A. McClelland, and M. Kaleko.** 1996. Sustained expression of therapeutic levels of human factor VIII in mice. *Blood 87:4671.*

16. **Connelly, S., J. L. Andrews, A. M. Gallo, D. B. Kayda, J. Qian, L. Hoyer, M. J. Kadan, M. I. Gorziglia, B. C. Trapnell, A. McClelland, and M. Kaleko.** 1998. Sustained phenotypic correction of murine hemophilia A by in vivo gene therapy. *Blood 91:3273.*

17. **Connelly, S., J. Mount, A. Mauser, J. M. Gardner, M. Kaleko, A. McClelland, and C. D. Lothrop, Jr.** 1996. Complete short-term correction of canine hemophilia A by in vivo gene therapy. *Blood 88:3846.*

18. **Dai, Y., E. M. Schwarz, D. Gu, W. W. Zhang, N. Sarvetnick, and I. M. Verma.** 1995. Cellular and humoral immune responses to adenoviral vectors containing factor IX gene: tolerization of factor IX and vector antigens allows for long-term expression. *Proc Natl Acad Sci U S A 92:1401.*

19. **Poller, W., S. Schneider-Rasp, U. Liebert, F. Merklein, P. Thalheimer, A. Haack, R. Schwaab, C. Schmitt, and H. H. Brackmann.** 1996. Stabilization of transgene expression by incorporation of E3 region genes into an adenoviral factor IX vector and by transient anti-CD4 treatment of the host. *Gene Ther 3:521.*

20. **Stein, C. S., J. L. Pemberton, N. van Rooijen, and B. L. Davidson.** 1998. Effects of macrophage depletion and anti-CD40 ligand on transgene expression and redosing with recombinant adenovirus. *Gene Ther 5:431.*

21. **Koeberl, D. D., I. E. Alexander, C. L. Halbert, D. W. Russell, and A. D. Miller.** 1997. Persistent expression of human clotting factor IX from mouse liver after intravenous injection of adeno-associated virus vectors. *Proc Natl Acad Sci U S A 94:1426.*

22. **Nakai, H., R. W. Herzog, J. N. Hagstrom, J. Walter, S. H. Kung, E. Y. Yang, S. J. Tai, Y. Iwaki, G. J. Kurtzman, K. J. Fisher, P. Colosi, L. B. Couto, and K. A. High.** 1998. Adeno-associated viral vector-mediated gene transfer of human blood coagulation factor IX into mouse liver. *Blood 91:4600.*

23. **Snyder, R. O., C. Miao, L. Meuse, J. Tubb, B. A. Donahue, H. F. Lin, D. W. Stafford, S. Patel, A. R. Thompson, T. Nichols, M. S. Read, D. A. Bellinger, K. M. Brinkhous, and M. A. Kay.** 1999. Correction of hemophilia B in canine and murine models using recombinant adeno-associated viral vectors [see comments]. *Nat Med 5:64.*

24. **Wang, L., K. Takabe, S. M. Bidlingmaier, C. R. Ill, and I. M. Verma.** 1999. Sustained correction of bleeding disorder in hemophilia B mice by gene therapy. *Proc Natl Acad Sci U S A 96:3906.*

25. **Herzog, R. W., J. N. Hagstrom, S. H. Kung, S. J. Tai, J. M. Wilson, K. J. Fisher, and K. A. High.** 1997. Stable gene transfer and expression of human blood coagulation factor IX after intramuscular injection of recombinant adeno-associated virus. *Proc Natl Acad Sci U S A 94:5804.*

26. **Katsumi, A., N. Emi, A. Abe, Y. Hasegawa, M. Ito, and H. Saito.** 1994. Humoral and cellular immunity to an encoded protein induced by direct DNA injection. *Hum Gene Ther 5:1335.*
27. **Herzog, R. W., E. Y. Yang, L. B. Couto, J. N. Hagstrom, D. Elwell, P. A. Fields, M. Burton, D. A. Bellinger, M. S. Read, K. M. Brinkhous, G. M. Podsakoff, T. C. Nichols, G. J. Kurtzman, and K. A. High.** 1999. Long-term correction of canine hemophilia B by gene transfer of blood coagulation factor IX mediated by adeno-associated viral vector. *Nat Med 5:56.*

11

CD4+ T CELLS SPECIFIC FOR FACTOR VIII AS A TARGET FOR SPECIFIC SUPPRESSION OF INHIBITOR PRODUCTION

Mark T. Reding[1,2], Huiyun Wu[1], Mark Krampf[1], David K. Okita[1], Brenda M. Diethelm-Okita[1], Nigel S. Key[2], and Bianca M. Conti-Fine[1,3,4]

Department of Biochemistry, Molecular Biology, and Biophysics[1], Department of Medicine[2], and Department of Pharmacology[3], University of Minnesota, Minneapolis-St. Paul, MN.

[4]Previously known as Bianca M. Conti-Tronconi

Supported by the NHLBI grant HL61922 (to B.M.C.-F.) and a research grant from the Hemophilia Association of New York (to N.S.K. and B.M.C.-F.). M.T.R. is the recipient of a Judith Graham Pool Postdoctoral Research Fellowship from the National Hemophilia Foundation.

INTRODUCTION

Some hemophilia A patients, when treated with factor VIII (fVIII) products to control bleeding episodes, develop antibodies (Ab) to surface domains of fVIII that are essential for its procoagulant function **(1-3)**. Development of fVIII inhibitors is a serious therapeutic complication that affects 20 – 25% of patients with hemophilia A **(1-3)**. Individuals without congenital fVIII deficiency may also develop pathogenic autoimmune inhibitory Ab to fVIII that cause acquired hemophilia, a rare yet severe bleeding disorder **(4,5)**. FVIII inhibitors are high affinity IgG, and their synthesis requires the intervention of fVIII specific CD4+ T helper cells.

Over the last several years, our laboratory has extensively investigated the role of CD4+ T cells in the pathogenesis of another Ab mediated disease, myasthenia gravis (MG). MG is an autoimmune neurological condition characterized by weakness that affects the ocular and other muscles innervated by the cranial nerves, and also limb muscles in most cases **(6)**. The symptoms of MG are caused by autoantibodies (autoAb) directed against the muscle nicotinic acetylcholine receptor (AChR) **(7)**. The ultimate goal of those studies was to lay the foundation for development of antigen-specific immunosuppressive treatments of the autoimmune response that causes MG, targeted on the antigen-specific CD4+ cells. More recently, we have begun investigating the characteristics and role(s) of fVIII specific CD4+ T cells in the development of fVIII inhibitors in both congenital and acquired hemophilia. We have also studied the presence of fVIII specific CD4+ T cells in healthy subjects, and have started to investigate the immune response to human fVIII in a murine model of hemophilia A.

Although they have no common clinical characteristics, the complications of hemophilia A management caused by inhibitors and the symptoms of MG share the same pathogenic mechanism—they are both caused by an undesirable Ab response. Also, in both conditions the pathogenic Ab are directed against well identified self antigens, of which we know the amino acid sequence, and many structural and functional properties. In both conditions the target self antigens are available in purified form. In both conditions the synthesis of the pathogenic Ab, which are high affinity IgG, requires intervention of CD4+T helper cells. Thus, it can be expected that similar investigative approaches may prove useful in understanding the mechanisms that lead to formation of the pathogenic autoAb in MG, and of inhibitors in hemophilia A. Also, it can be expected that both conditions could be corrected by "homologous" immunosuppressive strategies. Lastly, the availability of mouse models for both hemophilia A and MG makes it possible to carry out mechanistic studies on the pathogenesis of these conditions, and to test the efficacy of specific immunosuppressive treatments.

ROLE OF CD4+ T CELLS IN ANTIBODY SYNTHESIS

Antigen specific CD4+ T cells play a crucial role in humoral immune responses. Protein antigens are endocytosed by "professional" antigen presenting cells (APC) (i.e. cells such as macrophages and dendritic cells that are able to prime naive CD4+ T cells), denatured, and nicked by proteolytic enzymes. This releases from the antigen short linear peptide sequences, that are then bound by MHC class II molecules and exposed on the APC surface. CD4+ T cells recognize the antigen peptide/class II molecule complex **(8)**, whose engagement with the T cell antigen receptor leads to several events, including: 1) clonal expansion of T cells, mediated by autocrine interleukin (IL)-2 production; 2) differentiation of activated T cells into effector T cells; and 3) initiation of effector functions such as the secretion of cytokines which promote and regulate the humoral immune response (e.g., the synthesis of inhibitor antibodies) **(9)**.

In addition to antigen recognition, costimulatory pathways are required to achieve full physiologic activation of CD4+ T cells. For example, the T cell surface molecule CD28 binds to costimulatory molecules B7-1 (CD80) and B7-2 (CD86) expressed on the surface of APC. CD28 in turn promotes the activation of CD4+ T cells through mechanisms which are incompletely understood, yet essential for maximal CD4+ T cell activation **(10)**.

Activated B cells can also function as APC. Because they have surface membrane-bound immunoglobulin of the same antigen specificity as the Ab that they secrete, B cells are especially effective at processing and presenting epitope sequences derived from the same antigen recognized by the Ab they synthesize. The epitope/class II complexes on the B cell surface will be recognized by antigen-specific CD4+ cells, resulting in preferential cooperation between B cells and CD4+ T helper cells that recognize the same antigen (cognate T/B recognition) **(11)**.

ROLE OF Th1 AND Th2 CELLS IN THE IMMUNE RESPONSE

CD4+ T cells comprise different types of cells, which differ in their function and the cytokines they secrete **(12-14)**. Th1 and Th2 cells are distinct subsets of CD4+ T cells. Th1 cells carry out effector functions of the immune system. They secrete pro-inflammatory cytokines, such as interferon-γ, tumor necrosis factor and IL-2, and may be cytotoxic. They also help synthesis of IgG subclasses that bind complement, such as IgG1 in humans and IgG2 in mice. Th2 cells secrete anti-inflammatory cytokines such as IL-4 and IL-10, and help synthesis of Ab that do not bind complement, such as IgE, as well as IgG4 in humans and its homologue in mice, IgG1. Thus, while Th1 cells have an essential role in mediating effector functions of the immune response—either directly by virtue of their cytotoxic ability, or indirectly by stimulating the synthesis of Ab which fix complement—Th2 cells and the cytokines they secrete have complex and sometimes contrasting functions. They carry out effector functions by secreting IL-4 and IL-10, which are growth and differentiation factors for B cells, and stimulate production of IgE and other non-complement fixing Ab. On the other hand, Th2 cells suppress the immune response by secreting anti-inflammatory cytokines, which include IL-4 and IL-10, that inhibit the function of both APC and Th1 cells.

In addition, Th2 cells may down regulate an immune response indirectly, because IL-4 may be a growth factor for modulatory CD4+ cells that secrete TGF-β (also referred to as Th3 cells) **(15,16; however, see 17)**. The TGF-β family of cytokines are potent immunomodulators **(15)** that polarize CD4+ responses towards a Th2 phenotype **(18-20)** and block the effects of IL-12 in the development of Th1 responses **(19,21,22)**. Th3 cells do not produce IL-4, and may depend upon Th2 cells for proliferative signals **(15,23)**. Thus, Th2 cells may indirectly down-regulate immune responses through the action of IL-4 on Th3 cells.

Most fVIII inhibitors in hemophilia A patients are IgG4 and IgG1 **(24,25)**. In humans these IgG subclasses are induced by Th2 and Th1 cells, respectively. We recently found that mice genetically deficient in fVIII also have anti-fVIII Ab that are IgG of subclasses homologous to human IgG4 and IgG1 **(26)**. Thus, both Th2 and Th1 cells are involved in inhibitor synthesis. Determination of the extent to which Th1 and Th2 subsets are involved in the immune response to fVIII will be an important step towards understanding the immunobiology of fVIII inhibitors, and guiding the therapeutic strategy aimed at suppressing inhibitor formation.

ANTIGEN SPECIFIC TOLERANCE

Immunologic unresponsiveness to a specific antigen (tolerance) prevents the development of unwanted immune responses to non-pathogenic or self-antigens. Tolerance is maintained through an interplay of several different mechanisms, including "central" mechanisms that operate during maturation of the immune system, and "peripheral" mechanisms that occur when mature lymphocytes encounter antigens under specific conditions in the peripheral tissues. Immune tolerance is therefore a dynamic process which is actively maintained throughout life, rather than one which is established and "frozen" during prenatal and neonatal life **(27,28)**.

The appearance of inhibitors in hemophilia A patients appears to result from a complex interplay of host-related and fVIII-related factors. The mechanisms that may lead to development of fVIII inhibitors have been reviewed recently **(29)**. Since the synthesis of anti-fVIII Ab depends upon the action of CD4+ T cells specific for fVIII, induction of immunologic tolerance of these T cells should be an effective mechanism to prevent inhibitor formation.

Nasal, oral, or subcutaneous administration of antigens or peptide epitopes can induce specific T cell tolerance. This occurs through different mechanisms, depending on the dose of antigen or epitopes used **(30-33)**. Low doses generate regulatory Th2 cells **(31-33)**, which may exert a modulatory activity through secretion of cytokines such as IL-4 and IL-10 that act on Th1 cells in topographic proximity, irrespective of their antigen specificity (antigen-driven bystander suppression) **(34)**. Low doses may also cause anergy or deletion of the Th1 cells specific for the antigen or epitope administered. In contrast, high doses of antigen or epitopes induce anergy **(32,33)** and/or apoptosis **(30,35)** of antigen-specific Th1 and Th2 cells. Because Th2 cells are resistant to activation-induced cell death mediated by Fas/Fas ligand signaling **(36,37)**, higher doses of antigen are required to inactivate Th2 cells compared with Th1 cells.

There are potential dangers associated with the nasal, oral, or subcutaneous administration of antigens or peptide antigen epitopes. Low doses of antigen may activate antigen-specific Th2 helper cells, which can stimulate B cells **(12,23,38,39)**. The administered antigen could also stimulate antigen-specific B cells, and subsequent Ab synthesis **(12,23,38,40,41)**. In either case, the result would be the formation of Ab directed against the administered antigen. If native antigen were used for these tolerization procedures, the Ab thus formed may exacerbate the clinical condition. This may have disastrous consequences, as shown in marmoset experimental autoimmune encephalomyelitis **(39)**.

Short peptide epitopes are much safer than the whole antigen for T cell tolerance procedures, because their use would lead to the formation of Ab specific for the denatured peptide(s) **(42-44)**. Peptide-specific Ab seldom cross-react with the cognate native antigen **(45)**, and should therefore not cause any deleterious effects.

CD4+ T CELLS RECOGNIZE UNIVERSAL EPITOPES

A finding that has important ramifications for the development of tolerization procedures to fVIII is the demonstration that in humans a few small regions of the sequence of an antigen may be recognized by the CD4+ cells of every subject, irrespective of HLA-class II haplotype **(46-51)**. These regions have been termed "universal" CD4+ epitopes. Universal CD4+ epitopes are also immunodominant, because they appear to sensitize a large number of CD4+ cells **(50-52)**. Work done in our laboratory and by others has demonstrated the presence of universal CD4+ T cell epitopes for protein antigens such as the muscle nicotinic AChR **(49)**, diphtheria toxoid (DTD) **(50)**, and tetanus toxoid (TTD) **(46-48,51)**.

By analogy, fVIII should also have universal CD4+ T cell epitopes. We recently found that the A3 domain is recognized with high frequency by human anti-fVIII CD4+ cells **(53)**. This supports the possibility that fVIII contains universal epitopes, and that some are within the A3 domain. Identification and synthesis of universal epitope sequences for fVIII would allow their use for tolerization procedures suitable for the treatment of established fVIII inhibitors, without the need to investigate the epitope repertoire recognized by the CD4+ cells in each patient. Furthermore, it may be possible to prevent inhibitor development in high risk individuals by the administration of these peptides in a manner that results in tolerization, rather than activation, of the CD4+ clones potentially reactive to fVIII sequences, prior to the first therapeutic exposure to fVIII in infancy. Studies done in our laboratory (described below) with murine experimental myasthenia gravis (EMG) lend support to the idea that this approach may be successful in the management of fVIII inhibitors.

STRUCTURAL FEATURES OF UNIVERSAL CD4+ EPITOPES

The molecular basis for the existence of "universal" CD4+ epitopes is not known. Residues that flank those forming the "core" of the determinant may modulate the immunogenicity of a T epitope **(54)**. Such effects might be related to structural properties that permit proteolytic cleavage. Thus, certain sequences may be especially effective at sensitizing CD4+ cells because they might be easily processed and released from the antigen **(50,55)**. This, and the promiscuous binding of human class II molecules to peptides **(56-58)**, may result in their universal recognition by CD4+ cells.

We have intensely studied the epitopes recognized by human CD4+ cells on two model protein antigens, TTD and DTD, and we have identified several sequence regions that form universal, immunodominant epitopes **(50-52)**. The crystal structures of DTD **(59)**, of the receptor binding fragment H_C of tetanus neurotoxin **(60)**, and of botulinum neurotoxin **(61)**, which is highly homologous to tetanus neurotoxin, have been solved. This has allowed us to examine the structural features of the universal CD4+ epitopes and their flanking sequence regions.

All the sequence segments of DTD and TTD forming universal epitopes included, or were flanked by, residues forming relatively unstructured loops fully exposed to the solvent. Thus, solvent exposure of the end or flanking regions of a peptide sequence is a common feature of universal epitopes, that may be related to their immunodominance, because those exposed regions would be easily accessible targets for the proteolytic enzymes involved in antigen processing.

Another structural feature that might predict universal T cell epitopes is the local mobility within a protein antigen **(55)**. This might result in localized protease sensitivity and immunodominance of the sequence fragments released most easily. To determine whether the data obtained for the CD4+ epitope repertoire on TTD and DTD support the hypothesis that flexible segments direct antigen processing, we have compared the sequence location of the universal CD4+ epitopes with dynamic properties of the solved structures of DTD, of the fragment H_C of TTD, and botulinum toxin **(52)**. Crystallographic B factors, which weight the atom contribution in the calculation of electronic density from the model structure, are good indicators of the motility of the atoms in the crystal. High B factors correspond to weak density; that is, to poorly ordered atoms in the crystal. Analysis of the B factor of the α carbons is especially meaningful, because they should be the atoms that best reflect the motility of the peptide backbone. Sequence segments with high relative B factors were included in, and/or flanked one or both ends of all of the universal CD4+ epitopes identified on TTD and DTD, that in general aligned with "valleys" in the relative B factor values **(50-52)**.

The presence of solvent exposed sequence loops, and of sequence regions with high local mobility flanking the epitopes studied on TTD and DTD support the notion that immunodominance is influenced and facilitated by high protease sensitivity in the sequence loops flanking those epitopes. The crystal structure of the C2 domain of fVIII has been solved **(62)**, and that of the other domains is actively pursued. Furthermore, the crystal structure of ceruloplasmin, a serum protein structurally related to fVIII, has already been solved **(63)**. Identification of a few universal epitopes along a sequence of a protein as large as fVIII is a daunting task. The identification of the structural features discussed above as predictors of sequence regions that may form universal CD4+ epitopes, and the knowledge of the dynamic properties of the solved structures of fVIII or homologous proteins, may assist in the selection of sequence regions upon which to focus mapping efforts.

MURINE EXPERIMENTAL MYASTHENIA GRAVIS: A MODEL FOR SPECIFIC IMMUNOSUPPRESSION OF PATHOGENIC ANTIBODY RESPONSES

Murine EMG can be induced in C57Bl/6 (B6) mice by immunization with acetylcholine receptor (AChR) purified from the electric organ of *Torpedo californica*, and is a useful model for the study of Ab-mediated autoimmune diseases **(7)**. As in human MG, AChR-specific CD4+ T cells drive B cells to synthesize high affinity anti-AChR IgG Ab, resulting in a similar clinical phenotype **(7)**.

Using the murine EMG model, our laboratory has demonstrated that nasal or subcutaneous administration of synthetic peptide epitope sequences strongly recognized by AChR-specific CD4+ cells prevented the appearance of clinical symptoms after immunization with AChR **(42,43)**. The nasal or subcutaneous tolerization treatments also resulted in: 1) decreased CD4+ T cell responsiveness to the epitopes administered, and to the intact AChR, and 2) decreased synthesis of anti-AChR Ab **(42,43)**. The mechanisms involved in the protective effects of these procedures included anergy or deletion of Th1 cells and activation of down regulatory Th2 cells, resulting in a global suppression of the anti-AChR immune response, including synthesis of AChR-specific Ab. Administration of a limited number of AChR CD4+ epitope sequences, or even of just one immunodominant CD4+ epitope of the AChR , sufficed to block development of the Ab response against this antigen **(42,43)**.

This experimental system also illustrated the dangers of attempting to induce antigen-specific tolerization by the use of the complete antigen molecule, in contrast with the safety of using short peptide sequences. When AChR epitope peptides were administered to mice nasally or subcutaneously, the mice produced anti-peptide Ab that were not pathogenic **(42-44)**. Even prolonged subcutaneous treatment with the peptide epitopes did not worsen EMG symptoms **(43)**. On the other hand, subcutaneous treatment with solubilized AChR reduced the appearance of EMG symptoms when started before the immunization procedure, but it made the symptoms worse and more frequent when administered only after the appearance of EMG **(43)**. This suggests that subcutaneous administration of soluble AChR prior to immunization with this antigen reduced the priming of pathogenic AChR-specific immune cells, but administration following such priming stimulated the synthesis of pathogenic Ab. These results underline the potential dangers of the use of native autoantigen for tolerization procedures that may stimulate the synthesis of pathogenic Ab.

Further studies using IL-4 knock out mice, that have effective Th1 function yet severely impaired Th2 function **(64)**, have helped to clarify the important role that activation of modulatory Th2 cells have in the protective effect of tolerization procedures such as those described above. Those studies demonstrated that while sensitization of Th1 cells was sufficient to cause EMG, nasal administration of synthetic AChR epitopes which prevented development of EMG in B6 mice failed to do so in IL-4 knock out mice **(44)**. Although anergy or deletion of Th1 cells occurred in the peptide treated IL-4 knock out mice, this did not suffice to protect them from EMG or reduce the synthesis of anti-AChR antibodies **(44)**. Thus, the reduction in synthesis of anti-AChR Ab observed in wild type B6 mice after nasal or subcutaneous administration of AChR peptide epitopes must be mediated, directly or indirectly, by activation of peptide-specific regulatory Th2 cells.

The experiments in mouse EMG do not exclude the possibility that the protective effects of nasal and subcutaneous procedures are due to modulatory cytokines (e.g., TGF-β) secreted by Th3 cells. Those modulatory CD4+ cells could be specifically activated by the administered peptides, in the presence of IL-4 secreted by Th2 cells that were also activated by nasal or subcutaneous peptide administration.

Induction of tolerance in Th1 cells alone might prevent the development of pathogenic Ab, but this would require the use of a full complement of peptide epitope sequences that would be recognized by all of the pathogenic Th1 clones, and in doses sufficient to induce anergy or deletion of each specific Th1 clone. However, the activation of regulatory Th2 or Th3 cells specific for a few, or even one, immunodominant epitope could down regulate the immune response to the entire cognate antigen through the secretion of cytokines such as IL-4, IL-10 and TGF-β, that act on all Th1 cells in topographic proximity, regardless of their epitope specificity (antigen-driven bystander suppression) **(34)**. In addition, Th2 determinant spreading may occur **(65)**, and explain how sensitization of Th2 cells to an individual epitope might protect from an autoimmune disease that involves the entire cognate autoantigen.

ROLE OF CD4+ T CELLS IN THE DEVELOPMENT OF FVIII INHIBITORS

Successful induction of antigen-specific T cell tolerance requires that antigen-specific CD4+ cells are present in all patients, and that they are crucial for symptom development. Several lines of evidence point to the importance of the role of CD4+ T cells in the pathogenesis of fVIII inhibitors. Spontaneous disappearance of fVIII inhibitors can occur in HIV infected hemophiliacs in conjunction with the disease-related decline of CD4+ T cell counts **(66)**. The demonstration of increased IL-2 production by the peripheral blood mononuclear cells of patients with hemophilia following exposure to fVIII **(67)** suggests the involvement of T cells in the production of inhibitor Ab. T cell enriched peripheral blood mononuclear cells from hemophilia patients have also been shown to proliferate in response to fVIII **(68)** and fVIII specific T cells were demonstrated in the blood of some hemophilia A patients with inhibitors **(68,69)**. More recently, we have found that CD4+ cells that respond to fVIII are present in the blood of virtually all hemophilia patients **(53;** also, see below**)**. Finally, blockade of the B7/CD28 costimulatory pathway prevented development of anti-fVIII Ab in the murine model of hemophilia A **(70)**, providing direct evidence that the Ab response to fVIII is T cell dependent.

CD4+ T CELL RESPONSE TO FVIII IN HEMOPHILIA PATIENTS

To assess whether an approach similar to that described above will be feasible for the treatment of fVIII inhibitors, the epitope repertoire, phenotype (i.e., Th1, Th2, etc), and functional characteristics of fVIII-specific CD4+ T cells must be examined and defined. We have therefore undertaken a series of experiments designed to characterize the CD4+ T cell response to fVIII in patients with congenital and acquired hemophilia A **(53)**.

To facilitate a detailed study of the CD4+ epitope repertoire, we synthesized a library of peptides, each 20 residues long and overlapping by 10 residues, which spanned the entire fVIII sequence of 2332 amino acids **(71)**. The peptide length compared with that of naturally processed MHC class II restricted peptide epitopes **(72-74)**, and the overlapping nature of our peptide library reduced the risk of missing epitopes "broken" between peptides. We grouped synthetic peptides into pools corresponding to the sequence of individual fVIII domains (A1, A2, B, A3, C1, C2) (hereafter referred to as "fVIII domain pools"), and used them as representative antigens of the fVIII domains.

We have studied patients with acquired hemophilia, with severe hemophilia A and inhibitors, and with severe hemophilia A without inhibitors. Each month, for up to seven months, we tested the proliferative response of their blood CD4+ cells to intact recombinant fVIII and the fVIII domain pools described above. All patients had a significant CD4+ T cell response to fVIII at most of the time points tested. In all patients, the intensity of the CD4+ T cell response to fVIII fluctuated over time: most of them had one or more brief (one month) periods when we could not detect a response to fVIII. The overall characteristics of the response were similar in all three patient groups, each of which contained patients with vigorous and persistent responses, and patients with consistently low responses.

Most patients recognized most or all of the synthetic fVIII domain pools. Both hemophilia A and acquired hemophilia patients recognized domain A3 most commonly. The intensity of the responses to the domain pools correlated with that of the response to fVIII at the same point in time. Similar to the CD4+ T cell response to fVIII, the responses to the fVIII domain pools fluctuated in intensity over time. For most patients, the response to one or more of the fVIII domain pools occasionally decreased to undetectable levels for brief periods of time.

The patterns of fVIII domain recognition we observed in hemophilia patients did not correspond exactly to the location of the known major inhibitor binding epitopes within the A2, A3, and C2 domains **(75-78)**. Different considerations reconcile this discrepancy. First, Ab and T cell epitopes are seldom formed by the same sequence segments, since Ab recognize three dimensional epitopes on the surface of protein antigens, formed by amino acid residues that in most cases are within discontinuous sequence regions **(79)**, whereas T cells recognize short linear peptide sequences derived from the denatured, processed antigen **(80,81)**. Second, we have examined the responses of *all* anti-fVIII CD4+ T cells, not just the CD4+ T cells that preferentially help the synthesis of anti-fVIII Ab inhibitors. Anti-fVIII Ab may recognize domains that are functionally silent

(82,83): clearly in this case, the CD4+ cells that help their synthesis may recognize epitopes within domains other than those recognized by inhibitors.

HEALTHY SUBJECTS HAVE CD4+ T CELLS THAT RESPOND TO FVIII

The described presence of anti-fVIII Ab in healthy people **(84-86)**, suggests that fVIII-specific CD4+ cells may be sensitized without production of clinically significant anti-fVIII Ab. CD4+ cells that recognize self antigens, including autoantigens that are targets of pathogenic autoimmune responses, have been demonstrated frequently in healthy subjects **(87-94)**. Not all potentially self reactive T cells are deleted during ontogenesis of the immune system: given the characteristics of T cell epitopes, and their "simple" structure (short linear sequences comprising only a few residues), purging of all potentially self reactive T cells would reduce the T cell repertoire to a crippling extent, and make the immune system unable to deal with the broad universe of all possible exogenous T cell epitopes.

In addition, the "danger" theory of tolerance **(27)** predicts that the immune response discriminates not only on the basis of self and non self, but also whether an antigen is perceived as potentially dangerous or not. Thus, self proteins that are presented to CD4+ T cells in a context of "danger" (i.e., by professional APC at the site of an inflammatory reaction) will activate a response of the CD4+ T cells specific for that antigen, that had escaped clonal deletion. Serum proteins, including fVIII, may be especially prone to sensitize CD4+ cells. In healthy subjects, this may occur following extravasation of blood at hemorrhagic sites such as bruises, where an inflammatory reaction occurs, and epitope sequences from the extravasated fVIII and serum proteins may be presented by APC able to prime autoreactive CD4+ T cells specific for those epitopes. A report which describes the elution of a fVIII-derived peptide from purified human DR molecules **(95)** supports the notion that fVIII is commonly processed and presented in the human immune system.

We have undertaken a series of experiments, similar to those described above for the hemophilia patients, to determine whether healthy subjects also have CD4+ T cells that respond to fVIII, and to characterize such CD4+ responses **(53)**. We tested the blood CD4+ cells from twelve healthy subjects for their proliferative response to fVIII at approximately monthly intervals for up to sixteen months. In several experiments, we also tested the response to the fVIII domain pools.

All subjects had transient, yet significant and at times vigorous CD4+ T cell responses to fVIII. Overall, their responses were lower in intensity than those seen in the hemophilia patients. The intensity of the responses to fVIII also fluctuated over time, and the periods of non-reactivity tended to be more frequent, and longer than in hemophilia patients. Disappearance of fVIII specific CD4+ cells in healthy subjects is likely due to peripheral mechanisms of tolerance in the presence of the high normal blood levels of fVIII, that may cause inactivation of sensitized anti-fVIII CD4+ cells by anergy or apoptosis, following presentation of fVIII epitopes in the absence of costimulatory signals **(96-99).** The activated anti-fVIII CD4+ cells may persist for longer periods of time in hemophilia A patients because their low levels of fVIII, even after periodic replacement therapy, are not sufficient to sustain persistent tolerization of autoreactive CD4+ cells. In hemophilia A, the propensity to develop a CD4+ T cell response to fVIII is likely compounded by the abundance of potentially autoreactive CD4+ clones specific for fVIII, that were not deleted during ontogenesis of the immune system because of the absence of fVIII.

The findings described above and the relatively frequent presence of anti-fVIII Ab in healthy people **(84-86)** argue that development of clinically significant anti-fVIII Ab in hemophilia patients is due to inadequate mechanisms of tolerization of a normal immune response to fVIII, rather than—or in addition to—abnormal or excessive sensitization of CD4+ T cells to fVIII.

All healthy subjects responded to one or more fVIII domain pools in most experiments. In most subjects, a period of strong reactivity to one or more of the domain pools was either preceded or followed by periods of relatively little or no response to the same domain pools.

Like for the hemophilia patients, the A3 domain pool was recognized frequently. The finding that the A3 domain is recognized with high frequency in all patient groups and also in healthy subjects suggests that fVIII contains universal epitopes, and that some of them are within the A3 domain. A peptide previously found to be commonly bound to human MHC class II molecules also corresponds to residues 1775-1790 of the A3 domain **(95).** The identification of universal epitope sequences for fVIII would greatly facilitate the design of tolerization procedures aimed at suppressing or preventing inhibitor formation.

SUMMARY

The studies we reviewed here have begun to clarify the complex cellular mechanisms involved in the immune response to fVIII, and the circumstances under which fVIII inhibitors develop. Further characterization and comparison of the immune response to fVIII in both hemophilia patients and healthy subjects will help to further elucidate these mechanisms. The murine hemophilia model will hopefully provide further insights into the mechanisms of inhibitor formation, and prove to be a suitable tool for the design and testing of therapeutic strategies aimed at preventing the development of fVIII inhibitors.

REFERENCES

1. Aledort L. Inhibitors in hemophilia patients: Current status and management. Am J Hematol 1994; 47:208-217.

2. Hoyer LW. The incidence of factor VIII inhibitors in patients with severe hemophilia A. In: Aledort LM, Hoyer LW, Lusher JM, Reisner HM, White GC, eds. Inhibitors to Coagulation Factors. Adv Exp Med Biol 1995; 386:35-45.

3. Kreuz W, Escuriola-Ettingshausen C, Martinez-Saguer I, Gungor T, Kornhuber B. Epidemiology of inhibitors in haemophilia A. Vox Sang 1996; 70(suppl 1):2-8.

4. Shulman NR, Hirschman RJ. Acquired hemophilia. Trans Assoc Am Physicians 1969; 82:388-397.

5. Cohen AJ, Kessler CM. Acquired inhibitors. Baillieres Clin Haematol 1996; 9:331-354.

6. Engel AG. Myasthenia gravis and myasthenic syndromes. Ann Neurol 1984; 16:519-534.

7. Conti-Fine BM, Protti MP, Bellone M, Howard Jr. JF. Myasthenia gravis: The immunobiology of an autoimmune disease. RG Landes, Austin, 1997.

8. Germain RH, Margulies DM. The biochemistry and cell biology of antigen processing and presentation. Ann Rev Immunol 1993; 11:403-450.

9. Abbas AK, Lichtman AH, Pober JS. T lymphocyte antigen recognition and activation. In: Cellular and Molecular Immunology. Abbas AK, Lichtman AH, Pober JS, eds. Philadelphia: W.B. Saunders 1997; 138-170.

10. Lenschow DJ, Walunas TL, Bluestone JA. CD28/B7 system of T cell costimulation. Ann Rev Immunol 1996; 14:233-258.

11. Lanzavecchia K. Antigen-specific interaction between T and B cells. Nature 1985; 11:537-539.

12. Abbas A, Murphy K, Sher A. Functional diversity of helper T lymphocytes. Nature 1996; 383:787-793.

13. Romagnani S. The Th1/Th2 paradigm. Immunol Today 1997; 18:263-266.

14. Weigle WO, Romball CG. CD4+ T-cell subsets and cytokines involved in peripheral tolerance. Immunol Today 1997; 18:533-538.

15. O'Garra A, Steinman L, Gijbels K. CD4+ T cell subsets in autoimmunity. Curr Opin Immunol 1997; 9:872-883.

16. Seder RA, Mart T, Sieve MC, Strober W, Letterio J, Roberts AB, Kelsall B. Factors involved in the differentiation of TGF-β-producing cells from naïve CD4+ T cells: IL-4 and IFN-γ have opposing effects, while TGF-β positively regulates its own production. J Immunol 1998; 160:5719-5728.

17. Shi HN, Grusby MJ, Nagler-Anderson C. Orally induced peripheral nonresponsiveness is maintained in the absence of functional Th1 or Th2 cells. J Immunol 1999; 162:5143-5148.

18. Briere F, Servet-Delprat C, Bridon JM, Saint-Remy JM, Banchereau J. Human interleukin-10 induces naïve surface immunoglobulin D+ (sIgD+)B cells to secrete IgG1 and IgG3. J Exp Med 1994; 179:757-762.

19. Letterio J, Roberts AB. Regulation of immune responses by TGF-β. Ann Rev Immunol 1998; 16:137-161.

20. King C, Davies J, Mueller R, Lee MS, Krahl T, Yeung B, O'Connor E, Sarvetnick N. TGF-β1 alters APC preference, polarizing islet antigen responses toward a Th2 phenotype. Immunity 1998; 8:601-613.

21. Gorham JD, Guler ML, Fenoglio D, Gubler U, Murphy KM. Low dose TGF-β attenuates IL-12 responsiveness in murine Th cells. J Immunol 1998; 161:1664-1670.

22. Bright JJ, Sriram S. TGF-β inhibits IL-12-induced activation of Jak-STAT pathway in T lymphocytes. J Immunol 1998; 161:1772-1777.

23. O'Garra A. Cytokines induce the development of functionally heterogenous T helper cell subsets. Immunity 1998; 8:275-283.

24. Gilles JGG, Jacquemin MG, Saint-Remy JMR. Factor VIII inhibitors. Thromb Haemost 1997; 78:641-646.

25. Hoyer LW, Scandella D. Factor VIII inhibitors: Structure and function in autoantibody and hemophilia A patients. Semin Hematol 1994; 31(suppl 4):1-5.

26. Wu H, Krampf M, Karachunski PI, Okita DK, Reding MT, Lollar P, Hoyer LW, Conti-Fine BM. Hemophilia A mice treated with human factor VIII as a model system for formation of inhibitors. (manuscript in preparation)

27. Matzinger P. Tolerance, danger, and the extended family. Ann Rev Immunol 1994; 12:991-1045.

28. Nossal G. Choices following antigen entry: antibody formation or immunologic tolerance? Ann Rev Immunol 1995; 13:1-27.

29. Jacquemin MG, Saint-Remy JMR. Factor VIII immunogenicity. Haemophilia 1998; 4:552-557.

30. Chen Y, Inobe J, Marks R, Gonnella P, Kuchroo V, Weiner H. Peripheral deletion of antigen-reactive T cells in oral tolerance. Nature1995; 376:177-180.

31. Chen Y, Inobe J, Kuchroo V, Baron J, Janeway CJ, Weiner H. Oral tolerance in myelin basic protein T-cell receptor transgenic mice: suppression of autoimmune encephalomyelitis and dose-dependent induction of regulatory cells. Proc Natl Acad Sci USA 1996; 93:388-391.

32. Friedman A, Weiner HL. Induction of anergy or active suppression following oral tolerance is determined by antigen dosage. Proc Natl Acad Sci USA 1994; 91:6688-6692.

33. Gregerson D, Obritsch W, Donoso L. Oral tolerance in experimental autoimmune uveoretinitis. Distinct mechanisms of resistance are induced by low dose vs. high dose feeding protocols. J Immunol 1993; 151:5751-5761.

34. Weiner HL, Friedman A, Miller A, Khoury SJ, Al-Sabbagh, A, Santos L, Sayegh M, Nussenblatt RB, Trenthan DE, Hafler AD. Oral tolerance: immunologic mechanisms and treatment of animal and human organ-specific autoimmune diseases by oral administration of autoantigens. Ann Rev Immunol 1994; 12:809-837.

35. Critchfield JM, Racke MK, Zuniga-Pflucker JC, Cannella B, Rainse CS, Goverman J, Lenardo M. T cell deletion in high antigen dose therapy of autoimmune encephalomyelitis. Science 1994; 263:1139-1143.

36. Vardhachary AS, Perdow SN, Hu C, Ramanarayanan M, Salgame P. Differential ability of T cell subsets to undergo activation-induced cell death. Proc Natl Acad Sci USA 1997; 94:5778-5783.

37. Zhang X, Brunner T, Carter L, Dutton RW, Rogers P, Bradley L, Sato T, Reed JD, Green D, Swain SL. Unequal death in T helper cell (Th)1 and Th2 effectors: Th1, but not Th2, effectors undergo rapid Fas/FasL-mediated apoptosis. J Exp Med 1997; 185:1837-1849.

38. Neutra M, Pringult E, Kraehenbuhl J. Antigen sampling across epithelial barriers and induction of mucosal immune response. Ann Rev Immunol 1996; 14:275-300.

39. Genain CP, Abel K, Belmar N, Villinger F, Rosenberg DP, Linington C, Raine CS, Hauser SL. Late complications of immune deviation therapy in a non-human primate. Science 1996; 274:2054-2057.

40. Liu L, MacPherson GG. Antigen acquisition by dendritic cells: intestinal dendritic cells acquire antigen administered orally and can prime naïve T-cells in vivo. J Exp Med 1993; 177:1299-1307.

41. Husby S, Mestecky J, Moldoveanu Z, Holland S, Elson C. Oral tolerance in humans: T-cell but not B-cell tolerance after antigen feeding. J Immunol 1994; 152:4663-4670.

42. Karachunski P, Ostlie N, Okita D, Conti-Fine BM. Protection from experimental myasthenia gravis in C57Bl/6 mice by sniffing of synthetic CD4+ T cells epitopes. J Clin Invest 1997; 100:3027-3035.

43. Karachunski PI, Ostlie NS, Okita DK, Garman R, Conti-Fine BM. Subcutaneous administration of T-epitope sequences of the acetylcholine receptor prevents experimental myasthenia gravis. J Neuroimmunol 1999; 93:108-121.

44. Karachunski PI, Ostlie NS, Okita DK, Conti-Fine BM. Interleukin-4 deficiency facilitates developmemt of experimental myasthenia gravis and precludes its prevention by nasal administration of CD4+ epitope sequences of the acetylcholine receptor. J Neuroimmunol 1999; 95:73-84.

45. Conti-Fine BM, McLane KE, Lei S. Antibodies as tools to study the structure of membrane proteins: the case of the nicotinic acetylcholine receptor. Ann Rev Biophys Biomol Struct 1996; 25:197-229.

46. Panina-Bordignon P, Tan A, Termijtelen A, Demotz S, Corradin G, Lanzavecchia A. Universally immunogenic T cell epitopes: promiscuous binding to human MHC class II and promiscuous recognition by T cells. Eur J Immunol 1989; 19:2237-2242.

47. Ho PC, Mutch DA, Winkel KD, Saul AJ, Jones GL, Doran, TJ, Rzepczyk CM. Identification of two promiscuous T cell epitopes from tetanus toxin. Eur J Immunol 1990; 20:477-483.

48. Reece JC, Geysen HM, Rodda SJ. Mapping the major human T helper epitopes of tetanus toxin. The emerging picture. J Immunol 1993; 151:6175-6184.

49. Protti MP, Manfredi AA, Horton BM, Bellone M, Conti-Tronconi BM. Myasthenia Gravis: recognition of a human autoantigen at the molecular level. Immunol Today 1993; 14:363-368.

50. Raju R, Navaneethan D, Okita DK, Diethelm-Okita B, McCormick D, Conti-Fine BM. Epitopes for human CD4+ T cells on diphtheria toxin: structural features of sequence segments forming epitopes recognized by most subjects. Eur J Immunol 1995; 25:3207-3214.

51. Diethelm B, Raju R, Okita DK, Conti-Fine BM. Epitope repertoire of human CD4+ T cells on tetanus toxoid: identification of immunodominant sequence segments. J Infect Dis 1997; 175:382-391.

52. Diethelm-Okita BM, Okita DK, Banaszak L, Conti-Fine BM. Universal epitopes for human CD4+ cells on tetanus and diphtheria toxin. (submitted)

53. Reding MT, Wu H, Krampf M, Okita DK, Diethelm-Okita BM, Christie BA, Key NS, Conti-Fine BM. CD4+ T cell response to coagulation factor VIII in congenital and acquired hemophilia, and in healthy subjects. (submitted)

54. Moudgil KD, Sercarz EE, Grewal IS. Modulation of the immunogenicity of antigenic determinants by their flanking residues. Immunol Today 1998; 19:217-220.

55. Landry SJ. Local protein instability predictive of helper T-cell epitopes. Immunol Today 1997; 11:527-523.

56. Watts C. Capture and processing of exogenous antigens for presentation on MHC molecules. Ann Rev Immunol 1997; 15:821-850.

57. Madden DR. The three-dimensional structure of peptide-MHC complexes. Ann Rev Immunol 1995; 13:587-622.

58. Cresswell P. Assembly, transport, and function of MHC class II molecules. Ann Rev Immunol 1994; 12:259-294.

59. Choe S, Bennett MJ, Fujii G, Curmi PMG, Kantardjieff KA, Collier RJ, Eisenberg D. The crystal structure of diphtheria toxin. Nature 1992; 357:216.

60. Umland TC, Wingert LM, Swaminathan S, Furey WF, Schmidt JJ, Sax M. Srtucture of the receptor binding fragment H_c of tetanus neurotoxin. Nature Struct Biol 1997; 4:788-792.

61. Lacy DB, Tepp W, Cohen AC, DasGupta BR, Stevens RC. Crystal structure of botulinum neurotoxin type A and implications for toxicity. Nature Struct Biol 1998; 5:898-902.

62. Pellequer JL, Gale AJ, Griffin JH, Getzoff ED. Homology models of the C domains of blood coagulation factors V and VIII: a proposed membrane binding mode for FV and FVIII C2 domains. Blood Cells Mol Dis 1998; 24:448-461.

63. Pemberton S, Lindley P, Zaitsev V, Card G, Tuddenham EG, Kemball-Cook G: A molecular model for the triplicated A domains of human factor VIII based on the crystal structure of human ceruloplasmin. Blood 1997; 89:2413-2421.

64. Kuhn R, Rajewsky K, Muller W. Generation and analysis of interleukin-4 deficient mice. Science 1991; 254:707-710.

65. Tian J, Lehmann PV, Kaufman D. Determinant spreading of T helper cell 2 (Th2) responses to pancreatic islet autoantigens. J Exp Med 1997; 186:2039-2043.

66. Bray GL, Kroner BL, Arkin S, Aledort LW, Hilgartner MW, Etster ME, Ragni MV, Goedert JJ. Loss of high-responder inhibitors in patients with severe hemophilia A and human immunodeficiency virus type 1 infection: A report from the multi-center hemophilia cohort study. Am J Hematol 1993; 42:375-379.

67. Madhok R, Smith J, Jenkins A, Lowe GDO. T cell sensitization to factor VIII in hemophilia A? Br J Haematol 1991; 79:235-238.

68. Singer ST, Addiego Jr. JE, Reason DC, Lucas AH. T lymphocyte proliferative responses induced by recombinant factor VIII in hemophilia A patients with inhibitors. Thromb Haemost 1996; 76:17-22.

69. Newton-Nash DK, Gill JC, Foster PA: Cellular immune responses to coagulant factor VIII in F.VIII inhibitor patients, in Aledort LM, Hoyer LW, Lusher JM, Reisner HM, White GC, (eds): Inhibitors to Coagulation Factors. Adv Exp Med Biol 1995; 386:285.

70. Qian J, Collins M, Hoyer LW. Prevention of factor VIII inhibitors in murine hemophilia. Blood 1998 (abstr); 92(10):709a.

71. Vehar GA, Keyt B, Eaton D, Rodriguez H, O'Brien DP, Rotblat F, Oppermann H, Keck R, Wood WI, Harkins RN, Tuddenham EGD, Lawn RM, Capon DJ. Structure of human factor VIII. Nature 1894; 312:337-342.

72. Rudensky AY, Preston-Hurburt P, Hong SC, Barlow A, Janeway CA Jr. Sequence analysis of peptide bound to MHC class II molecules. Nature 1991; 353:622-627.

73. Hunt DF, Michel H, Dickison TA, Shabanowitz J, Cox AL, Sakaguchi K, Appella E, Grey HM, Sette A. Peptides presented to the immune system by the murine class II major histocompatibility complex molecule I-A^d. Science 1992; 256:1817-1820.

74. Stern LJ, Brown JH, Jardetzky TS, Gorga JC, Urban RG, Strominger JL, Wiley DC. Crystal structure of the human class II MHC protein HLA-DR1 complexed with an influenza virus peptide. Nature 1994; 368:215-221.

75. Scandella D, Gilbert GE, Shima M, Nakai H, Eagleson C, Felch M, Prescott R, Rajalakshmi KJ, Hoyer LW, Saenko E: Some factor VIII inhibitor antibodies recognize a common epitope corresponding to C2 domain amino acids 2248 through 2312, which overlap a phospholipid-binding site. Blood 1995; 86:1811-1819.

76. Shima M, Nakai H, Scandella D, Tanaka I, Sawamoto Y, Kamisue S, Morichika S, Murakami T, Yoshioka A: Common inhibitory effects of human anti-C2 domain inhibitor alloantibodies on factor VIII binding to von Willebrand factor. Br J Haematol 1995; 91:714-721.

77. Healey JF, Lubin IM, Nakai H, Saenko E, Hoyer LW, Scandella D, Lollar P: Residues 484-508 contain a major determinant of the inhibitory epitope in the A2 domain of human factor VIII. J Biol Chem 1995; 270:14505-14509.

78. Zhong D, Saenko EL, Shima M, Felch M, Scandella D: Some human inhibitor antibodies interfere with factor VIII binding to factor IX. Blood 1998; 92:136-142.

79. Davies DR, Cohen GH: Interactions of protein antigens with antibodies. Proc Natl Acad Sci USA 1996; 93:7-12.

80. Engelhard VH: Structure of peptides associated with class I and class II molecules. Annu Rev Immunol 1994; 12:181-207.

81. Garcia KC, Teyton L, Wilson IA: Structural basis of T cell recognition. Annu Rev Immunol 1999; 17:369-397.

82. Nilsson IM, Berntorp E, Zettervall O, Dahlback B: Noncoagulation inhibitory factor VIII Ab after induction of tolerance to factor VIII in hemophilia A patients. Blood 1990; 75:378-383.

83. Gilles JGG, Arnout J, Vermylen J, Saint-Remy J-MR: Anti-factor VIII Ab of hemophiliac patients are frequently directed towards nonfunctional determinants and do not exhibit isotypic restriction. Blood 1993; 82:2452-2461.

84. Batlle J, Gomez E, Rendal E, Torea J, Loures E, Couselo M, Vila P, Sedano C, Tusell X, Magallon M, Quintana M, Gonzalez-Boullosa R, Lopez-Fernandez MF: Ab to factor VIII in plasma of patients with hemophilia A and normal subjects. Ann Hematol 1996; 72:321-326.

85. Gilles JG, Saint-Remy J-MR: Healthy subjects produce both anti-factor VIII and specific anti-idiotypic antibodies. J Clin Invest 1994; 94:1496-1505.

86. Algiman M, Dietrich G, Nydegger UE, Boieldieu D, Sultan Y, Kazatchkine MD: Natural Ab to factor VIII (anti-hemophilic factor) in healthy individuals. Proc Natl Acad Sci USA 1992; 89:3795-3799.

87. Moiola L, Karachunski P, Protti M, Howard J, Conti-Tronconi BM. Epitopes on the ß suounit of muscle acetylcholine receptor recognized by CD4+ cells of myasthenia patients and healthy subjects. J Clin Invest 1994; 93:1020-1028.

88. Kellerman S, McCormick D, Freeman S, Morris J, Conti-Fine BM. TSH receptor sequences recognized by CD4+ cells in Graves' disease patients and in healthy controls. J Autoimmunity 1995; 8:685-698.

89. Burns J, Rosenzweig A, Zweiman B, Lisak RP. Isolation of myelin basic protein-reactive T-cell lines from normal human blood. Cell Immunol 1983; 81:435-440.

90. Pette M, Fujita K, Wilkinson D, Altmann DM, Trowsdale J, Giegerich G, Hinkkanen A, Epplen JT, Kappos L, Wekerle H. Myelin autoreactivity in multiple sclerosis: Recognition of myelin basic protein in the context of HLA-DR2 products by T lymphocytes of multiple sclerosis patients and healthy donors. Proc Natl Acad Sci USA 1990; 87:7968-7972.

91. Ota K, Matusi M, Milford EL, Mackin GA, Weiner HL, Hafler DA. T-cell recognition of an immunodominant myelin basic protein epitope in multiple sclerosis. Nature 1990; 346:183-187.

92. Kuwana M, Medsger TA Jr, Wright TM. T cell proliferative response induced by DNA topoisomerase I in patients with systemic sclerosis and healthy donors. J Clin Invest 1995; 96:586-596.

93. Ito Y, Nieda M, Uchigata Y, Nishimura M, Tokunaga K, Kuwata S, Obata F, Tadokoro K, Hirata Y, Omori Y, Juji T. Recognition of human insulin in the context of HLA-DRB1*0406 products by T cells of insulin autoimmune syndrome patients and healthy donors. J Immunol 1993; 151:5770-5776.

94. Hoffman RW, Takeda Y, Sharp GC, Lee DR, Hill DL, Kaneoka H, Caldwell CW. Human T cell clones reactive against U-small nuclear ribonucleoprotein autoantigens from connective tissue disease patients and healthy individuals. J Immunol 1993; 151:6460-6469.

95. Chicz RM, Urban RG, Gorga JC, Vignali DAA, Lane WS, Strominger JL: Specificity and promiscuity among naturally processed peptides bound to HLA-DR alleles. J Exp Med 1993; 178:27-47.

96. Fisher GH, Rosenberg FJ, Straus SE, Dale JK, Middleton LR, Lin RY, Strober W, Lenardo MJ, Puck JM: Dominant interfering Fas gene mutations impair apoptosis in a human autoimmune lymphoproliferative syndrome. Cell 1995; 81:935-946.

97. Rieux-Laucat F, Le Deist F, Hivroz C, Roberts IR, Debatin KM, Fisher A, de Villartay JP: Mutations in Fas associated with human lymphoproliferative syndrome and autoimmunity. Science 1995; 268:1347-1349.

98. Johnson JG, Jenkins MK: The role of anergy in peripheral T cell unresponsiveness. Life Sci 1994; 55:1767-1780.

99. Schwartz RH: Models of T cell anergy: Is there a common molecular mechanism? J Exp Med 1996; 184:1-8.

12

CD40L PATHWAY BLOCKADE AS AN APPROACH TO IMMUNOTHERAPY

Linda C. Burkly
Biogen, Inc.

INTRODUCTION

CD154, also known as CD40 Ligand (CD40L), was discovered in 1992 as the ligand for CD40. Initial studies of this pathway generated great excitement as these coreceptors were recognized as the long sought after molecular mediators of cognate T cell help for B cells. This seminal finding was the culmination of efforts begun decades prior by Mitchison and others, when cell-cell cooperation was first shown to be required for the elicitation of antibody (Ab) production in response to protein antigens (ags) (1). Although identified recently, progress in dissecting the role of the pathway in normal physiologic and pathologic processes has been rapid and provocative. Herein is a concise overview of the pivotal role of the CD40L pathway in regulating humoral and cell-mediated immunity (CMI), and its more recently discovered role in events underlying fibrosis and vascular pathology. The potential for therapeutic application of CD40L blockade is emphasized. In particular, promising results of recent experiments in nonhuman primate model systems with a humanized anti-CD40L mAb, humanized 5C8 (hu5C8) are summarized. CD40L-dependent and CD40L-independent immunity are discussed, providing basis for the favorable activity profile observed in animals treated with this powerful immunomodulatory approach.

EXPRESSION OF CD154 (CD40L) AND CD40

CD154, also known as gp39 (2, 3), TBAM (4, 5), TRAP (6), and CD40L (7), is a member of the Tumor Necrosis Factor (TNF) superfamily (8). CD40L is a 39 kD Type II transmembrane protein which forms a heterotrimer on the cell surface (9), homologous to other ligands such as TNF, Lymphotoxin (LT)α, LTβ, and FasL. TNF, discovered in the early 1900's, is the prototypic member of this continually expanding family of molecules. TNF family members are broadly recognized for their key roles in promoting inflammation, triggering cell death, and regulating the neogenesis and organization of peripheral lymphoid organs, reviewed in (8, 10, 11). The addition of CD40L to this family based on structural homology, ultimately evidenced at crystallographic level (12), was initially surprising given the functional significance of CD40L in promoting immune cell activation and enhancing cell survival.

CD40L is characterized by an activation-dependent, temporally restricted expression pattern. This molecule is primarily expressed on T helper (T_H) cells

Hemophilia Care in the New Millennium, edited by D. Monroe *et al.*
Kluwer Academic/Plenum Publishers, 2001

transiently after activation through the T cell receptor (TcR). CD40L reaches peak level expression by 4-6 hours post-activation and declines rapidly after 16-18 hours (5, 6, 13). The transient nature of CD40L expression after ag triggering makes this molecule an attractive target for selective modulation of immune responses. In addition to $CD4^+$ T cells, CD40L has been reported to be expressed by other cell types after activation *in vitro*, though the physiological significance of all of these findings are not clear at this time. These include a subset of $CD8^+$ T cells (14), basophils and mast cells (15), eosinophils (16), natural killer (NK) cells (17), B cells (18, 19), macrophages (mϕ) (20) and dendritic cells (DC) (21). Recently, CD40L also has been shown to be expressed on the surface of activated platelets (22).

CD40, the counter-receptor for CD40L, is a member of the TNF-receptor superfamily (23). CD40 was first discovered in 1989 (24) as a critical molecule for B cell activation based on the induction of B cell proliferation by CD40 crosslinking by mAbs (25-27). CD40 is a 45-50kDa Type I integral membrane protein which is multimerized by engagement of CD40L. Essentially, each CD40 molecule binds to a CD40L trimer at the molecular interface formed by two monomers. In this way, three CD40 molecules engage one molecule of CD40L. The CD40 receptor has a broad distribution pattern, (28). CD40 is constitutively expressed on the surface of B cells, mϕ, DC and thymic epithelium. Interestingly, within the last two years, CD40 also has been reported at very low levels on the surface of many different nonhematopoeitic cells types, including epithelial cells, mesenchymal cells such as fibroblasts (FB) and smooth muscle cells (SMC), and endothelial cells (EC) (29-37). Furthermore, these reports demonstrate that this low level CD40 expression is markedly increased by exposure to IFNγ. As such, it is

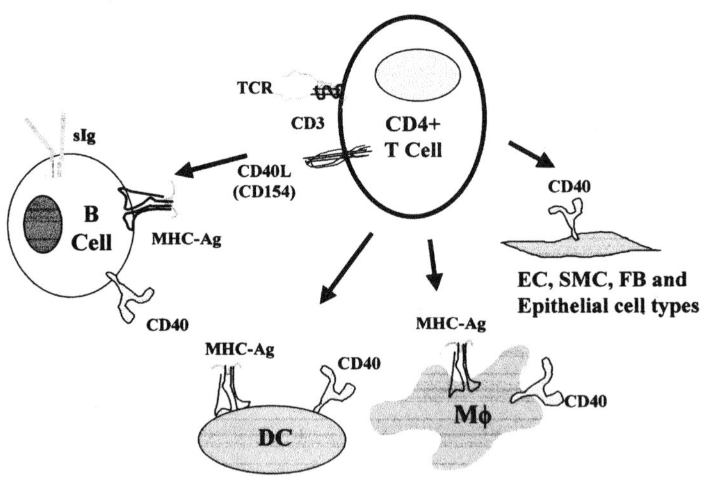

Figure 1. Key cellular interactions mediated by the CD40L/CD40 pathway. Activated $CD40L^+$ T_H cells interact with $CD40^+$ B cells, dendritic cells (DC), macrophages (mϕ), endothelial cells (EC), smooth muscle cells (SMC), fibroblasts (FB) and epithelial cells to induce multiple immune and inflammatory mechanisms.

now apparent that the key cellular interactions and functions mediated by the CD40L/CD40 pathway encompass areas of biology which include humoral and CMI, as well as fibrosis and vascular biology (see Figure 1).

ROLE OF CD40L IN T_H CELL COSTIMULATION

Immune responses are orchestrated by a critical subset of ag-reactive T lymphocytes, $CD4^+$ T_H cells. Each T_H cell bears TcR which recognize a specific ag-derived peptide in the cleft of a Class II Major Histocompatibility Complex (MHC) molecule presented on the surface of antigen presenting cells (APC). DC, mϕ and B cells all may serve as APC. T_H cells also express a variety of molecules on their surface which serve to stabilize their interaction with APC by binding to their counter-receptors expressed on APC. These include LFA-1, VLA-4 and CD2 on the T cell side binding to ICAM-1, VCAM-1 and LFA-3, respectively (38, 39). Ag recognition by T_H cells is coupled to signal transduction through the TcR thereby initiating T_H cell activation.

Other T cell surface molecules also may transmit signals upon engaging their ligands expressed on APC, "costimulating" with the TcR to achieve optimal T_H cell activation. Such costimulatory pathways include the CD2/LFA-3 and CD28/B7 systems (39-41). In particular, when B7-1 or B7-2 expressed on activated APC engage the CD28 molecule on T cells, a key "second signal" is transmitted. T cells are costimulated to express bcl-2 and IL-2 which promote T cell survival and expansion, respectively. The CD40L/CD40 pathway is another such costimulatory pathway. There is some evidence that a signal may be transmitted through CD40L (42-44). However, this aspect is still unresolved. On the other hand, it is well accepted that the CD40L pathway mediates T cell costimulation through its regulation of B7-1 and B7-2 expression. The B7 molecules are low or absent on APC prior to their interaction with T_H cells. These molecules are significantly upregulated by signals transmitted through CD40 (45) subsequently stimulating T_H cells through CD28. Thus CD40L initiates a cascade of reciprocal activation events, resulting in APC activation and optimal T_H cell priming (46, 47), and reviewed in (48, 49).

In addition to upregulating activation molecules on the surface of APC, the CD40L pathway is responsible for the induction and regulation of multiple immune effector mechanisms, (50). As outlined above, after primary activation through the TcR, the T_H cell expresses CD40L, physically interacts with $CD40^+$ accessory cell types, and delivers signals through the CD40 receptor. T_H cells promote humoral immunity through their interaction with B cells. Consequently, B cell differentiation leads to the generation of Ab-secreting cells and memory B cells. $CD40L^+$ T_H cells interact with mϕ and DC, promoting CMI through activation of these cell types and through the generation of natural killer cells (NK cells) and cytotoxic T lymphocytes (CTL).

Thus the CD40L/CD40 pathway distinguishes itself from other costimulatory pathways through its role as a master switch, playing a pivotal role in regulating the function of T_H cells as well as many aspects of accessory cell function. The critical function of the CD40L pathway in mediating cross-talk between T_H cells and accessory cells is depicted in Figure 2.

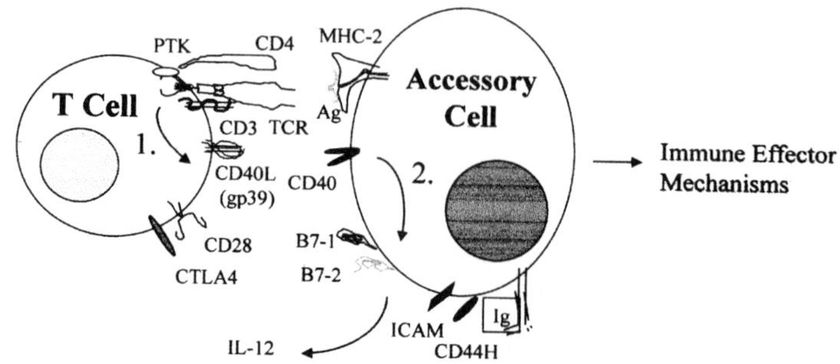

Figure 2. The CD40L pathway mediates T_H cell priming through the induction of costimulatory molecule expression and cytokine production by APC. In particular, B7-1 and B7-2 costimulate T_H cells through CD28, and IL-12 acts on T_H cells to promote differentiation to the T_{H1} cell type.

ROLE OF CD40L IN THE INDUCTION OF IMMUNE EFFECTOR MECHANISMS: ACTIVATION OF CD40$^+$ HEMATOPOEITIC CELLS AND CD40$^+$ STROMAL CELL TYPES

Initial studies of the CD40L/CD40 pathway identified it as cognate mediator of B cell activation by T_H cells *in vitro* (2, 5, 51), and reviewed in (28). The contribution of genetic approaches was key to this understanding. The discovery that human subjects with hyper-IgM syndrome carried mutations in the CD40L gene revealed that CD40L was responsible for their defective Ab production and failure to switch from IgM to IgG in response to ags (52). These functions also have been extensively dissected in genetically engineered mice with disrupted CD40L or CD40 gene loci, CD40L (53, 54) and CD40 (55, 56) knockout mice, respectively, and through the use of blocking Abs specific for this molecule. It is now well recognized that signals through CD40 are required for B cell proliferation and differentiation leading to the generation of Ab producing cells *in vivo* (57, 58). In addition, CD40L is required for the formation of germinal centers (GC), foci of antigen-reactive B cells induced to proliferate by antigen-specific T_H cells (53-56, 59). The processes occurring in GC and the molecular control of these events have been reviewed in detail (60, 61). GC B cells employ their Ig receptors to capture ag which has been trapped by local follicular DC. Competition for limited ag is based on Ig receptor affinity. B cells which effectively compete will process and present antigen to T_H cells, thereby receiving cooperative CD40L-dependent B cell survival signals (62, 63). In this way, proliferating B cells which have undergone mutations which improve Ig receptor affinity are selectively expanded (64). Other CD40L-dependent events which are critical to the maturation of the immune response also occur in GC, namely isotype switching from IgM to other Ig subclasses (64) and the generation of B cell memory (59, 65).

The role of the CD40L/CD40 pathway is well established for the generation of primary and secondary Ab responses, GC development and the generation of B cell memory. However, its role in humoral immunity after the initiation of a response and in the maintenance of memory requires further investigation. Pertinent to this issue, Han et al. showed that anti-CD40L mAbs administered to mice approximately one week after ag exposure dissolved GC that had already formed at that point (66). This result demonstrated that CD40L is required to maintain established GC. However, the effect of anti-CD40L mAb treatment on B cell memory under these conditions was not assessed. It is unknown whether the GC B cells were deleted or relocated elsewhere. Our experiments in nonhuman primates indicate that the CD40L pathway is not required to maintaim an ongoing immune response when anti-CD40L mAbs are administered six weeks after primary ag exposure. Specifically, monkeys treated with anti-CD40L mAb hu5C8 six weeks after immunization with tetanus toxoid (TT) ag maintained anti-TT titers that were comparable to those in control monkeys immunized with TT but not hu5C8-treated. By contrast, during the period of drug exposure, their response to another ag was significantly inhibited (Biogen Inc., unpublished observations). The extent to which the nature of the ag, the dose and the persistence influence the CD40L-dependence of humoral immunity also requires further investigation. These aspects are highly relevant to the potential success of CD40L blockade as a treatment for ongoing Ab-mediated autoimmune disorders. Thus far, available data from animal models are promising (see below).

The role of the CD40L pathway in eliciting CMI also was suggested through the phenotype of the hyperIgM patients who suffer from increased susceptibility to intracellular pathogens which are normally handled by T cell-activated mϕ, such as Pneumocystis carinii pneumonia and Cryptosporidium infections (67). This type of defect also has been observed in CD40L deficient mice (68). It is now established that CD40L delivers critical signals through CD40 on mϕ (69) and DC (70, 71) thereby enabling cell-mediated inflammatory responses (72). One of the key effector functions induced by CD40L is the production of proinflammatory cytokines by mϕ and DC, including TNF, IL-1 and IL-12 (73-76). IL-12 is particularly important as it is a powerful stimulus for differentiation of T_{H1} cells (77). This is a T_H cell type defined by secretion of a unique profile of cytokines including TNF, LTα and IFNγ which activate accessory cells. Thus CD40L/CD40 induced IL-12 stimulates a positive feedback loop between T_H and accessory cells, promoting and amplifying the cellular arm of the immune response.

More recently the ability of CD40L on T_H cells to enhance DC survival (78, 79) has been appreciated. This function effectively prolongs ag presentation to T cells, providing another example of the reciprocal cell activation triggered by the CD40L/CD40 pathway. As a result, effective priming of T_H cells occurs in response to soluble protein ags and foreign cell surface MHC molecules (alloantigens). In addition, CD40-activated DC effectively present ag to CD8+ T cells for the generation of CTL (80-82), a primary effector mechanism for the elimination of virally-infected cells and transplanted cells bearing alloantigens. Interestingly, virus-specific T_H cell and CTL responses can be elicited by alternative pathways (see below). However, the generation of alloantigen-reactive T_H cells and CTL are highly CD40L-dependent (83-86). Taken together, these support the application of CD40L blockade to treatment of T_{H1}-type autoimmune disease and prevention of transplant rejection.

The role of the CD40L pathway in regulating the function of nonhematopoeitic cell types is still a relatively new area of investigation. It is now clear that CD40L induces the expression of adhesion molecules such as ICAM-1 and VCAM-1 (31, 32), and production of pro-inflammatory cytokines and chemokines such as TNF, IL-1 and IL-8, MCP-1, RANTES, and MIP-1α by a variety of stromal cell types (32, 87-91). These include EC, FB, SMC and epithelial cells. These events likely occur in the context of an ongoing inflammatory process since activation through CD40 on these cells types requires or is augmented by prior to exposure to IFNγ. Thus the CD40L pathway regulates leukocyte migration to inflammatory sites through its effect on adhesion molecules and chemoattractants produced by stromal cells. In addition, CD40L induces fibroblast proliferation *in vitro* (32), making it a candidate pathway for the regulation of fibrosis *in vivo*. Consistent with the latter possibility, CD40 expression has been reported on nonhematopoeitic cell types in human renal tissue from glomerulonephritis patients (92). It is further supported by the results of studies showing that CD40L blockade can reduce kidney and spleen fibrosis in a murine model of systemic lupus erythematosis (SLE) (93) wherein anti-CD40L mAb treatment was initiated after establishment of disease, and in murine models of hyperoxic and radiation injury-induced lung fibrosis (94, 95).

Expression of CD40 also has been documented in the vessels of transplanted organs on EC (96) and by EC, SMC and mϕ in atherosclerotic lesions (35). These data suggest a role for the pathway in the interaction of CD40L$^+$ cells and vascular elements. CD40L$^+$ T_H cells or activated platelets could interact with vessels in a proinflammatory environment thereby promoting vascular fibrosis typical of acute and chronic graft rejection. In the setting of lipid-induced vascular injury, the CD40L pathway could promote processes underlying the progression of vascular lesions (35). This hypothesis is supported by the results of anti-CD40L treatment on atherogenesis in a murine atherosclerosis-prone strain (97). Still more recently, CD40L has been shown to induce metalloproteinase production by EC, SMC and mϕ, (98-101) and the formation of capillary tubules in fibrin matrix gels *in vitro* (102). This has prompted speculation regarding the role of CD40L in neovascularization settings. The physiological significance of these *in vitro* observations remains to be established, as there are no reported vascular defects in hyperIgM patients or in CD40L knockout mice, and prolonged CD40L blockade does not impair wound healing in surgical settings of transplantation in rodents or monkeys (103-105).

THERAPEUTIC ACTIVITY OF CD40L BLOCKADE IN RODENTS AND NONHUMAN PRIMATES

The central role of the CD40L pathway in regulating immune effector cells suggests a variety of potential therapeutic applications. This potential is clearly supported by the promising results of studies with anti-CD40L specific mAbs in an array of murine models. These findings are briefly summarized in Table 1 with accompanying references (83-86, 93-95, 97, 106-126). The studies by Kalled (93) and Howard et al. (111) are particularly exciting with respect to therapeutic potential of CD40L blockade. In these studies the therapeutic effects of the anti-CD40L mAb MR1 were demonstrated after disease establishment. In the murine SLE model (93), MR1 treatment of mice with established nephritis significantly decreased mortality and improved renal function, inhibiting kidney fibrosis and preventing increases in anti-double stranded DNA autoAb titers. Similarly, treatment with MR1 after the onset of clinical symptoms in a murine model of experimental allergic encephaomyelitis (EAE) resulted in significant improvement (111). Furthermore, MR1 treatment during remission of EAE inhibited the occurrence of clinical relapses.

Investigations in nonhuman primates also have been conducted in order to test this promising immunomodulatory approach in higher order species (summarized in Table 2). These experiments have been executed through the use hu5C8 which is reactive with human and nonhuman primate CD40L. Administration of hu5C8 to cynomolgus monkeys significantly inhibits the generation of primary and secondary Ab responses to foreign proteins (127), similar to observations made in mouse model systems. Notably, inhibition was similar in naive and in primed animals, with up to 80% inhibition of total TT-specific Ig titers.

Impressive data also has been obtained in numerous independent studies establishing the ability of hu5C8 to inhibit rejection of vascularized organ and islet allotransplants. The ability of hu5C8 monotherapy to significantly prolong acceptance of fully MHC-mismatched renal allografts was established in a rhesus monkey model wherein recipient animals had their native kidneys removed (128). In these experiments, graft rejection in untreated control animals occurred within eight days after transplant. By contrast, animals treated with hu5C8 as an induction therapy, ie. administered every few days over the course of the first two weeks post transplant, retained their grafts for about 100 postoperative days. Hu5C8 also effectively reversed acute, ongoing rejection episodes which occurred in the animals at that time. Similarly, hu5C8 has been shown to prolong the survival of heterotopic cardiac allografts in cynomolgus monkeys (129). The ability of hu5C8 to promote indefinite graft survival was further explored in the renal allograft model by continuing hu5C8 dosing after the induction phase, administering drug on a monthly basis for six months post transplant. The results recently reported show rejection-free allograft survival and stable function in 9/9 rhesus recipients, with three of them longer than 500 days post transplant (103). Strikingly, drug has been discontinued in three of these animals for as long as six months to a year. Thus the hu5C8 treatment appears to have induced a state wherein grafts are not rejected even after disappearance of drug from the circulation. The mechanism of action of hu5C8 is not fully understood at this time. However, it is apparent that the activation of accessory cells and effector mechanisms including CTL which play a prominent role in graft rejection have been abrogated. The fate of the alloantigen-reactive T cells in unclear, though possibly this antigen-reactive subset has been deleted or anergized. Interestingly, lymphocytic infiltrates including T cells confined to the interstitium of the graft were noted in the hu5C8 treated animals. In addition, certain generalized immunosuppressive agents which act to inhibit TcR signaling in alloantigen-specific T_H cells appeared to diminish the beneficial effects of hu5C8. Taken together, it is reasonable to speculate that the immunomodulatory effect of hu5C8 requires an active process. The fate of the alloantigen-specific T cells and the nature of the cellular infiltrates certainly requires further study.

The ability of hu5C8 to prevent allograft rejection also has been recently reported in a nonhuman primate models of islet cell transplantation (104, 105). The application of hu5C8 in this setting is particularly attractive since there is no currently approved drug regimen for islet transplantation. This setting is characterized by significant hurdles, namely allograft rejection and recurrent autoimmunity. In addition, many of the conventional immunosuppressive agents are inappropriate for this application since they impair islet function. In these reports, nonhuman primates rendered diabetic by complete pancreatectomy received intraportal islet transplants with or without hu5C8 treatment. Similar to the renal allograft study findings, hu5C8 induction therapy significantly prolonged islet allograft acceptance in treated baboons as measured by normal blood glucose levels and insulin independence (105). By comparison, recipients which were untreated or treated with a conventional immunosuppressive agent rejected their islets promptly within eight days. In addition, hu5C8 effectively reversed ongoing rejection episodes in these baboon recipients. The effect of continuing hu5C8 as a monthly maintenance therapy was further explored in rhesus monkey recipients (104). Islet engraftment and insulin independence was observed in 6/6 recipient animals, the longest followed for over 400 days post transplant. The effect of discontinued drug administration is reportedly in progress. However, it is most interesting that hu5C8 treated recipients became unresponsive to donor alloantigen as measured by *in vitro* mixed lymphocytes cultures (MLC) and remained responsive to third party cells. The powerful immunomodulatory effect of hu5C8 in these nonhuman primate model systems supports its potential application to prevent clinical transplant rejection and curb immunopathologies, including ongoing autoimmune diseases.

Table 1 Role of CD40L/CD40 Pathway in Murine Disease Models: Inhibitory Effects of Anti-CD40L mAb Treatment *in Vivo*

Models of Autoimmunity	Effect	References
Lupus Nephritis in genetically predisposed mice	Delayed spontaneous disease onset and reduced incidence when administered to pre-nephritic mice	106, 107
	Prolonged survival and improved renal function in mice with established nephritis; reduced kidney and spleen fibrosis	93
Insulin-Dependent Diabetes Mellitus in genetically predisposed mice	Prevented spontaneous diabetes when treatment was initiated during early stages of disease development; impaired TH1 cell priming	108
Collagen-induced Arthritis	Prevented disease induction, inhibiting joint inflammation and anti-collagen Ab production	109
Experimental Allergic	Prevented disease induc-	110

Table 1, continued

Encephalomyelitis	tion, also reduced clinical score when administered after disease onset	
	Reduced relapse rate in a relapsing-remitting model when given at peak of acute disease or during remission; inhibited TH1 differentiation	111
Induced-Oophoritis	Prevented disease induc- and antibody production to an ovarian glycoprotein epitope	112
TNBS-Induced Colitis	Prevented disease induction and inhibited production of IL-12	113
Model of Inflammation		
Acute Viral Myocarditis	Decreased myocardial inflammation induced by Coxsackievirus B3	114
Models of Allotransplantation	Effect	References
Graft vs. Host Disease (GVHD)	Blocked acute and chronic GVHD; inhibited donor anti-host allo-specific helper T cell and CTL responses	83-85
Cardiac, Liver, Aorta, Skin, Islet	Prevented or delayed graft rejection, in some cases in combination with donor-specific lymphocytes or CD28/B7 blockade	86, 115-126 (selected references)
Models of Fibrosis		
Hypertoxic-induced lung fibrosis	Reduced pulmonary injury	94, 95
Radiation-induced lung fibrosis	Improved survival and reduced lung pathology	
Model of Vascular Pathology		
Atherosclerosis in genetically predisposed mice	Limited size and lipid content of lesions in LDL receptor KO mice fed a high cholesterol diet	97

Table 2 Therapeutic Effect of Humanized anti-CD40L mAb hu5c8 in Nonhuman Primate Model Systems

Model	Effect	Reference
Antibody production	Inhibits primary and secondary antibody responses to tetanus toxoid	127
Renal allograft rejection	Prolongs renal allograft survival Reverses ongoing renal allograft rejection	128
Renal allograft rejection	Prevents renal allograft rejection Long-term survival after mAb therapy suspended	103
Cardiac allograft rejection	Prolongs cardiac allograft survival	129
Islet allograft rejection	Prolongs islet allograft survival Insulin independence achieved Reverses ongoing islet allograft rejection	105
Islet allograft rejection	Prevents islet allograft rejection Insulin dependence achieved	104

CD40L-INDEPENDENT IMMUNITY

Immune responses which are activated and regulated by T_H cells are said to be T_H-dependent whereas those which do not require T cell help are said to be T-independent (TI). Prototypic TI ags are polysaccharides. Due to their repetitive structures, these ags are able to highly crosslink ag-specific immunoglobulin (Ig) receptors on B cells and thereby trigger B cells without cognate T cell help. Given the polysaccharide-rich composition of bacteria, Ab production in response to these pathogens is largely TI. Thus CD40L blockade is not expected to impair protective immunity to bacteria or their components. Consistent with this, the CD40L-independence of carbohydrate ag responses has been directly demonstrated in CD40L knockout mice (53, 54). By contrast, the CD40L/ CD40 pathway is essential for many T_H-dependent responses. Although these generally include responses to soluble protein ags and to alloantigens, there are likely to be many factors which influence their dependence on CD40L. For example, the response to protein ags administered in adjuvant are more difficult to inhibit with anti-CD40L Abs, suggesting that the ability of adjuvants to directly activate accessory cells or costimulate T_H cells and thereby initiate the inflammatory cascade allows them to bypass CD40L. Alternatively, adjuvants may serve to increase ag dose by promoting persistence and thereby may decrease CD40L-dependence.

Viral infection is another antigenic stimulus that is relatively CD40L-independent (130). This is supported by observations made in mice demonstrating the CD40L independence of primary anti-viral responses, though memory CTL responses were somewhat CD40L-dependent (131-134). Significantly, hyperIgM patients show no increased risk of viral infection (67). The basis for the relative CD40L-independence of viral responses was revealed by an elegant experiment (81) indicating that viral infection directly activates DC, thereby enabling them to effectively present ag and induce virus-specific CTL without the need for costimulation . In addition, in cases where virus-specific T_H cells are involved, it appears that other pathways substitute for CD40L in priming of the virus-specific T_H cells. Namely, new coreceptors in the TNF/TNF-receptor family, designated Receptor Activator of NF-kB Ligand (RANKL), also called TRANCE, and its receptor RANK, have been shown to play a role in the priming virus-specific T_H cells (135-137) and reviewed in (138). In the Lymphocytic Choriomeningitis Virus (LCMV) system in mice, RANKL and CD40L compensate for each other as evidenced by the need to inhibit both pathways in order to effectively inhibit T_H priming (139). By contrast, the immune response to replication defective viral vectors such as those used for gene therapy applications appears to be more sensitive to inhibition by CD40L blockade (140-144).

In summary, the CD40L-dependence of immunity appears to be influenced by the properties of the ag. Based on experimental data in mice, bacterial and viral responses are expected to remain largely intact. Consistent with this, nonhuman primate study results indicate that anti-CD40L exposure is safe and well-tolerated as characterized by normal weight gain and good health status, with no increased incidence of bacterial or viral infection and no impairment in wound healing.

CLOSING REMARKS

The central role of the CD40L/CD40 pathway in regulating T_H -dependent immunity has been impressively dissected over the past seven years. Promising results indicating the therapeutic potential of this approach have been generated in both rodent and nonhuman primate model systems. These data support the clinical testing of CD40L blockade in autoimmune disease and transplantation settings. Further advances are required to better our understanding of the role of the pathway in regulating non-hematopoeitic cell function, and to define the mechanism of action of this approach to enable optimization of its application.

ACKNOWLEDGEMENTS

I would like to thank Dr. Paula Hochman for helpful suggestions while writing this review and Dr. Hochman and Dr. Susan Kalled for critical reading of this manuscript.

REFERENCES

1. Mitchison, N.A. 1967. *Cold Spring Harbor Symposium* 32:431.
2. Noelle, R.J., M. Roy, D.M. Shepherd, I. Stamenkovic, J.A. Ledbetter, and A. Aruffo. 1992. A 39-kDa protein on activated helper T cells binds CD40 and transduces the signal for cognate activation of B cells. *Proc Natl Acad Sci U S A* 89, no. 14:6550.
3. Hollenbaugh, D., L.S. Grosmaire, C.D. Kullas, N.J. Chalupny, S. Braesch-Andersen, R.J. Noelle, I. Stamenkovic, J.A. Ledbetter, and A. Aruffo. 1992. The human T cell antigen gp39, a member of the TNF gene family, is a ligand for the CD40 receptor: expression of a soluble form of gp39 with B cell co-stimulatory activity. *Embo J* 11, no. 12:4313.
4. Lederman, S., M.J. Yellin, G. Inghirami, J.J. Lee, D.M. Knowles, and L. Chess. 1992. Molecular interactions mediating T-B lymphocyte collaboration in human lymphoid follicles. Roles of T cell-B-cell-activating molecule (5C8 antigen) and CD40 in contact-dependent help. *J Immunol* 149, no. 12:3817.
5. Lederman, S., M.J. Yellin, A. Krichevsky, J. Belko, J.J. Lee, and L. Chess. 1992. Identification of a novel surface protein on activated CD4+ T cells that induces contact-dependent B cell differentiation (help). *J Exp Med* 175, no. 4:1091.
6. Graf, D., U. Korthauer, H.W. Mages, G. Senger, and R.A. Kroczek. 1992. Cloning of TRAP, a ligand for CD40 on human T cells. *Eur J Immunol* 22, no. 12:3191.
7. Armitage, R.J., W.C. Fanslow, L. Strockbine, T.A. Sato, K.N. Clifford, B.M. Macduff, D.M. Anderson, S.D. Gimpel, T. Davis-Smith, C.R. Maliszewski, and et al. 1992. Molecular and biological characterization of a murine ligand for CD40. *Nature* 357, no. 6373:80.
8. Gruss, H.J., and S.K. Dower. 1995. The TNF ligand superfamily and its relevance for human diseases. *Cytokines Mol Ther* 1, no. 2:75.
9. Hsu, Y.M., J. Lucci, L. Su, B. Ehrenfels, E. Garber, and D. Thomas. 1997. Heteromultimeric complexes of CD40 ligand are present on the cell surface of human T lymphocytes. *J Biol Chem* 272, no. 2:911.
10. Smith, C.A., T. Farrah, and R.G. Goodwin. 1994. The TNF receptor superfamily of cellular and viral proteins: activation, costimulation, and death. *Cell* 76, no. 6:959.
11. Chaplin, D.D., and Y. Fu. 1998. Cytokine regulation of secondary lymphoid organ development. *Curr Opin Immunol* 10, no. 3:289.
12. Karpusas, M., Y.M. Hsu, J.H. Wang, J. Thompson, S. Lederman, L. Chess, and D. Thomas. 1995. 2 A crystal structure of an extracellular fragment of human CD40 ligand. *Structure* 3, no. 12:1426.
13. Roy, M., T. Waldschmidt, A. Aruffo, J.A. Ledbetter, and R.J. Noelle. 1993. The regulation of the expression of gp39, the CD40 ligand, on normal and cloned CD4+ T cells. *J Immunol* 151, no. 5:2497.
14. Lane, P., A. Traunecker, S. Hubele, S. Inui, A. Lanzavecchia, and D. Gray. 1992. Activated human T cells express a ligand for the human B cell- associated antigen CD40 which participates in T cell-dependent activation of B lymphocytes. *Eur J Immunol* 22, no. 10:2573.
15. Gauchat, J.F., S. Henchoz, G. Mazzei, J.P. Aubry, T. Brunner, H. Blasey, P. Life, D. Talabot, L. Flores-Romo, J. Thompson, and et al. 1993. Induction of human IgE synthesis in B cells by mast cells and basophils. *Nature* 365, no. 6444:340.
16. Gauchat, J.F., S. Henchoz, D. Fattah, G. Mazzei, J.P. Aubry, T. Jomotte, L. Dash, K. Page, R. Solari, D. Aldebert, and et al. 1995. CD40 ligand is functionally expressed on human eosinophils. *Eur J Immunol* 25, no. 3:863.
17. Carbone, E., G. Ruggiero, G. Terrazzano, C. Palomba, C. Manzo, S. Fontana, H. Spits, K. Karre, and S. Zappacosta. 1997. A new mechanism of NK cell cytotoxicity activation: the CD40-CD40 ligand interaction. *J Exp Med* 185, no. 12:2053.
18. Grammer, A.C., M.C. Bergman, Y. Miura, K. Fujita, L.S. Davis, and P.E. Lipsky. 1995. The CD40 ligand expressed by human B cells costimulates B cell responses. *J Immunol* 154, no. 10:4996.
19. Wykes, M., J. Poudrier, R. Lindstedt, and D. Gray. 1998. Regulation of cytoplasmic, surface and soluble forms of CD40 ligand in mouse B cells. *Eur J Immunol* 28, no. 2:548.
20. Mach, F., U. Schonbeck, G.K. Sukhova, T. Bourcier, J.Y. Bonnefoy, J.S. Pober, and P. Libby. 1997. Functional CD40 ligand is expressed on human vascular endothelial cells, smooth muscle cells, and macrophages: implications for CD40-CD40 ligand signaling in atherosclerosis. *Proc Natl Acad Sci U S A* 94, no. 5:1931.
21. Pinchuk, L.M., S.J. Klaus, D.M. Magaletti, G.V. Pinchuk, J.P. Norsen, and E.A. Clark. 1996. Functional CD40 ligand expressed by human blood dendritic cells is up- regulated by CD40 ligation. *J Immunol* 157, no. 10:4363.

22. Henn, V., J.R. Slupsky, M. Grafe, I. Anagnostopoulos, R. Forster, G. Muller-Berghaus, and R.A. Kroczek. 1998. CD40 ligand on activated platelets triggers an inflammatory reaction of endothelial cells. *Nature* 391, no. 6667:591.

23. Baker, S.J., and E.P. Reddy. 1998. Modulation of life and death by the TNF receptor superfamily. *Oncogene* 17, no. 25:3261.

24. Stamenkovic, I., E.A. Clark, and B. Seed. 1989. A B-lymphocyte activation molecule related to the nerve growth factor receptor and induced by cytokines in carcinomas. *Embo J* 8, no. 5:1403.

25. Clark, E.A., and J.A. Ledbetter. 1986. Activation of human B cells mediated through two distinct cell surface differentiation angtigens, Bp35 and Bp50. *Proc. Natl. Acad. Sci. USA* 83:4494.

26. Gordon, J., M.J. Millsum, G.-R. Guy, and J.A. Ledbetter. 1987. Synergistic interaction between interleukin-4 and anti-Bp50 (CDw40) revealed in a novel B cell restimulation assay. *Eur. J. Immunol.* 17:1535.

27. Rousset, F., E. Garcia, and J. Banchereau. 1991. Cytokine-induced proliferation and immunoglobulin production of human B lymphocytes triggered through their CD40 antigen. *J Exp Med* 173, no. 3:705.

28. Banchereau, J., F. Bazan, D. Blanchard, F. Briere, J.P. Galizzi, C. van Kooten, Y.J. Liu, F. Rousset, and S. Saeland. 1994. The CD40 antigen and its ligand. *Annu Rev Immunol* 12:881.

29. Yellin, M.J., J. Brett, D. Baum, A. Matsushima, M. Szabolcs, D. Stern, and L. Chess. 1995. Functional interactions of T cells with endothelial cells: the role of CD40L-CD40-mediated signals. *J Exp Med* 182, no. 6:1857.

30. Hollenbaugh, D., N. Mischel-Petty, C.P. Edwards, J.C. Simon, R.W. Denfeld, P.A. Kiener, and A. Aruffo. 1995. Expression of functional CD40 by vascular endothelial cells. *J Exp Med* 182, no. 1:33.

31. Karmann, K., C.C. Hughes, J. Schechner, W.C. Fanslow, and J.S. Pober. 1995. CD40 on human endothelial cells: inducibility by cytokines and functional regulation of adhesion molecule expression. *Proc Natl Acad Sci U S A* 92, no. 10:4342.

32. Yellin, M.J., S. Winikoff, S.M. Fortune, D. Baum, M.K. Crow, S. Lederman, and L. Chess. 1995. Ligation of CD40 on fibroblasts induces CD54 (ICAM-1) and CD106 (VCAM- 1) up-regulation and IL-6 production and proliferation. *J Leukoc Biol* 58, no. 2:209.

33. Fries, K.M., G.D. Sempowski, A.A. Gaspari, T. Blieden, R.J. Looney, and R.P. Phipps. 1995. CD40 expression by human fibroblasts. *Clin Immunol Immunopathol* 77, no. 1:42.

34. Banchereau, J., B. Dubois, J. Fayette, N. Burdin, F. Briere, P. Miossec, M.C. Rissoan, C. van Kooten, and C. Caux. 1995. Functional CD40 antigen on B cells, dendritic cells and fibroblasts. *Adv Exp Med Biol* 378:79.

35. Mach, F., U. Schonbeck, and P. Libby. 1998. CD40 signaling in vascular cells: a key role in atherosclerosis? *Atherosclerosis* 137 Suppl:S89.

36. Wrone-Smith, T., T. Johnson, B. Nelson, L.H. Boise, C.B. Thompson, G. Nunez, and B.J. Nickoloff. 1995. Discordant expression of Bcl-x and Bcl-2 by keratinocytes in vitro and psoriatic keratinocytes in vivo. *Am J Pathol* 146, no. 5:1079.

37. Young, L.S., A.G. Eliopoulos, N.J. Gallagher, and C.W. Dawson. 1998. CD40 and epithelial cells: across the great divide. *Immunol Today* 19, no. 11:502.

38. Elangbam, C.S., C.W. Qualls, Jr., and R.R. Dahlgren. 1997. Cell adhesion molecules--update. *Vet Pathol* 34, no. 1:61.

39. Wingren, A.G., E. Parra, M. Varga, T. Kalland, H.O. Sjogren, G. Hedlund, and M. Dohlsten. 1995. T cell activation pathways: B7, LFA-3, and ICAM-1 shape unique T cell profiles. *Crit Rev Immunol* 15, no. 3-4:235.

40. Chambers, C.A., and J.P. Allison. 1999. Costimulatory regulation of T cell function. *Curr Opin Cell Biol* 11, no. 2:203.

41. McAdam, A.J., A.N. Schweitzer, and A.H. Sharpe. 1998. The role of B7 co-stimulation in activation and differentiation of CD4+ and CD8+ T cells. *Immunol Rev* 165:231.

42. Brenner, B., U. Koppenhoefer, H. Grassme, J. Kun, F. Lang, and E. Gulbins. 1997. Evidence for a novel function of the CD40 ligand as a signalling molecule in T-lymphocytes. *FEBS Lett* 417, no. 3:301.

43. Brenner, B., U. Koppenhoefer, A. Lepple-Wienhues, H. Grassme, C. Muller, C.P. Speer, F. Lang, and E. Gulbins. 1997. The CD40 ligand directly activates T-lymphocytes via tyrosine phosphorylation dependent PKC activation. *Biochem Biophys Res Commun* 239, no. 1:11.

44. Koppenhoefer, U., B. Brenner, F. Lang, and E. Gulbins. 1997. The CD40-ligand stimulates T-lymphocytes via the neutral sphingomyelinase: a novel function of the CD40-ligand as signalling molecule. *FEBS Lett* 414, no. 2:444.

45. Ranheim, E.A., and T.J. Kipps. 1993. Activated T cells induce expression of B7/BB1 on normal or leukemic B cells through a CD40-dependent signal. *J Exp Med* 177, no. 4:925.
46. Grewal, I.S., J. Xu, and R.A. Flavell. 1995. Impairment of antigen-specific T-cell priming in mice lacking CD40 ligand. *Nature* 378, no. 6557:617.
47. Grewal, I.S., H.G. Foellmer, K.D. Grewal, J. Xu, F. Hardardottir, J.L. Baron, C.A. Janeway, Jr., and R.A. Flavell. 1996. Requirement for CD40 ligand in costimulation induction, T cell activation, and experimental allergic encephalomyelitis. *Science* 273, no. 5283:1864.
48. Grewal, I.S., and R.A. Flavell. 1996. A central role of CD40 ligand in the regulation of CD4+ T-cell responses. *Immunol Today* 17, no. 9:410.
49. Mackey, M.F., R.J. Barth, Jr., and R.J. Noelle. 1998. The role of CD40/CD154 interactions in the priming, differentiation, and effector function of helper and cytotoxic T cells. *J Leukoc Biol* 63, no. 4:418.
50. van Kooten, C., and J. Banchereau. 1997. Functions of CD40 on B cells, dendritic cells and other cells. *Curr Opin Immunol* 9, no. 3:330.
51. Spriggs, M.K., R.J. Armitage, L. Strockbine, K.N. Clifford, B.M. Macduff, T.A. Sato, C.R. Maliszewski, and W.C. Fanslow. 1992. Recombinant human CD40 ligand stimulates B cell proliferation and immunoglobulin E secretion. *J Exp Med* 176, no. 6:1543.
52. Korthauer, U., D. Graf, H.W. Mages, F. Briere, M. Padayachee, S. Malcolm, A.G. Ugazio, L.D. Notarangelo, R.J. Levinsky, and R.A. Kroczek. 1993. Defective expression of T-cell CD40 ligand causes X-linked immunodeficiency with hyper-IgM [see comments]. *Nature* 361, no. 6412:539.
53. Xu, J., T.M. Foy, J.D. Laman, E.A. Elliott, J.J. Dunn, T.J. Waldschmidt, J. Elsemore, R.J. Noelle, and R.A. Flavell. 1994. Mice deficient for the CD40 ligand [published erratum appears in Immunity 1994 Oct;1(7):following 613]. *Immunity* 1, no. 5:423.
54. Renshaw, B.R., W.C. Fanslow, 3rd, R.J. Armitage, K.A. Campbell, D. Liggitt, B. Wright, B.L. Davison, and C.R. Maliszewski. 1994. Humoral immune responses in CD40 ligand-deficient mice. *J Exp Med* 180, no. 5:1889.
55. Kawabe, T., T. Naka, K. Yoshida, T. Tanaka, H. Fujiwara, S. Suematsu, N. Yoshida, T. Kishimoto, and H. Kikutani. 1994. The immune responses in CD40-deficient mice: impaired immunoglobulin class switching and germinal center formation. *Immunity* 1, no. 3:167.
56. Castigli, E., F.W. Alt, L. Davidson, A. Bottaro, E. Mizoguchi, A.K. Bhan, and R.S. Geha. 1994. CD40-deficient mice generated by recombination-activating gene-2- deficient blastocyst complementation. *Proc Natl Acad Sci U S A* 91, no. 25:12135.
57. Van den Eertwegh, A.J., R.J. Noelle, M. Roy, D.M. Shepherd, A. Aruffo, J.A. Ledbetter, W.J. Boersma, and E. Claassen. 1993. In vivo CD40-gp39 interactions are essential for thymus-dependent humoral immunity. I. In vivo expression of CD40 ligand, cytokines, and Ab production delineates sites of cognate T-B cell interactions. *J Exp Med* 178, no. 5:1555.
58. Foy, T.M., D.M. Shepherd, F.H. Durie, A. Aruffo, J.A. Ledbetter, and R.J. Noelle. 1993. In vivo CD40-gp39 interactions are essential for thymus-dependent humoral immunity. II. Prolonged suppression of the humoral immune response by an Ab to the ligand for CD40, gp39. *J Exp Med* 178, no. 5:1567.
59. Foy, T.M., J.D. Laman, J.A. Ledbetter, A. Aruffo, E. Claassen, and R.J. Noelle. 1994. gp39-Cd40 interactions are essential for germinal center formation and the development of B cell memory. *J Exp Med* 180, no. 1:157.
60. MacLennan, I.C. 1994. Germinal centers. *Annu Rev Immunol* 12:117.
61. Liu, Y.-J., and J. Banchereau. 1996. The paths and molecular controls of peripheral B-cell development. *The Immunologist* 4, no. 2:55.
62. Lagresle, C., P. Mondiere, C. Bella, P.H. Krammer, and T. Defrance. 1996. Concurrent engagement of CD40 and the antigen receptor protects naive and memory human B cells from APO-1/Fas-mediated apoptosis. *J Exp Med* 183, no. 4:1377.
63. Fang, W., K.A. Nath, M.F. Mackey, R.J. Noelle, D.L. Mueller, and T.W. Behrens. 1997. CD40 inhibits B cell apoptosis by upregulating bcl-xL expression and blocking oxidant accumulation. *Am J Physiol* 272, no. 3 Pt 1:C950.
64. Liu, Y.J., D.E. Joshua, G.T. Williams, C.A. Smith, J. Gordon, and I.C. MacLennan. 1989. Mechanism of antigen-driven selection in germinal centres. *Nature* 342, no. 6252:929.
65. Arpin, C., J. Dechanet, C. Van Kooten, P. Merville, G. Grouard, F. Briere, J. Banchereau, and Y.J. Liu. 1995. Generation of memory B cells and plasma cells in vitro. *Science* 268, no. 5211:720.
66. Han, S., K. Hathcock, B. Zheng, T.B. Kepler, R. Hodes, and G. Kelsoe. 1995. Cellular interaction in germinal centers. Roles of CD40 ligand and B7-2 in established germinal centers. *J Immunol* 155, no. 2:556.

67. Levy, J., T. Espanol-Boren, C. Thomas, A. Fischer, P. Tovo, P. Bordigoni, I. Resnick, A. Fasth, M. Baer, L. Gomez, E.A. Sanders, M.D. Tabone, D. Plantaz, A. Etzioni, V. Monafo, M. Abinun, L. Hammarstrom, T. Abrabamsen, A. Jones, A. Finn, T. Klemola, E. DeVries, O. Sanal, M.C. Peitsch, and L.D. Notarangelo. 1997. Clinical spectrum of X-linked hyper-IgM syndrome [see comments]. *J Pediatr* 131, no. 1 Pt 1:47.

68. Soong, L., J.C. Xu, I.S. Grewal, P. Kima, J. Sun, B.J. Longley, Jr., N.H. Ruddle, D. McMahon-Pratt, and R.A. Flavell. 1996. Disruption of CD40-CD40 ligand interactions results in an enhanced susceptibility to Leishmania amazonensis infection. *Immunity* 4, no. 3:263.

69. Alderson, M.R., R.J. Armitage, T.W. Tough, L. Strockbine, W.C. Fanslow, and M.K. Spriggs. 1993. CD40 expression by human monocytes: regulation by cytokines and activation of monocytes by the ligand for CD40. *J Exp Med* 178, no. 2:669.

70. Caux, C., C. Massacrier, B. Vanbervliet, B. Dubois, C. Van Kooten, I. Durand, and J. Banchereau. 1994. Activation of human dendritic cells through CD40 cross-linking. *J Exp Med* 180, no. 4:1263.

71. Flores-Romo, L., P. Bjorck, V. Duvert, C. van Kooten, S. Saeland, and J. Banchereau. 1997. CD40 ligation on human cord blood CD34+ hematopoietic progenitors induces their proliferation and differentiation into functional dendritic cells. *J Exp Med* 185, no. 2:341.

72. Stout, R.D., and J. Suttles. 1996. The many roles of CD40 in cell-mediated inflammatory responses. *Immunol Today* 17, no. 10:487.

73. Kiener, P.A., P. Moran-Davis, B.M. Rankin, A.F. Wahl, A. Aruffo, and D. Hollenbaugh. 1995. Stimulation of CD40 with purified soluble gp39 induces proinflammatory responses in human monocytes. *J Immunol* 155, no. 10:4917.

74. Shu, U., M. Kiniwa, C.Y. Wu, C. Maliszewski, N. Vezzio, J. Hakimi, M. Gately, and G. Delespesse. 1995. Activated T cells induce interleukin-12 production by monocytes via CD40-CD40 ligand interaction. *Eur J Immunol* 25, no. 4:1125.

75. Koch, F., U. Stanzl, P. Jennewein, K. Janke, C. Heufler, E. Kampgen, N. Romani, and G. Schuler. 1996. High level IL-12 production by murine dendritic cells: upregulation via MHC class II and CD40 molecules and downregulation by IL-4 and IL-10 [published erratum appears in J Exp Med 1996 Oct 1;184(4):following 1590]. *J Exp Med* 184, no. 2:741.

76. Cella, M., D. Scheidegger, K. Palmer-Lehmann, P. Lane, A. Lanzavecchia, and G. Alber. 1996. Ligation of CD40 on dendritic cells triggers production of high levels of interleukin-12 and enhances T cell stimulatory capacity: T-T help via APC activation. *J Exp Med* 184, no. 2:747.

77. Trinchieri, G. 1995. Interleukin-12: a proinflammatory cytokine with immunoregulatory functions that bridge innate resistance and antigen-specific adaptive immunity. *Annu Rev Immunol* 13:251.

78. Bjorck, P., J. Banchereau, and L. Flores-Romo. 1997. CD40 ligation counteracts Fas-induced apoptosis of human dendritic cells. *Int Immunol* 9, no. 3:365.

79. Ludewig, B., D. Graf, H.R. Gelderblom, Y. Becker, R.A. Kroczek, and G. Pauli. 1995. Spontaneous apoptosis of dendritic cells is efficiently inhibited by TRAP (CD40-ligand) and TNF-alpha, but strongly enhanced by interleukin- 10. *Eur J Immunol* 25, no. 7:1943.

80. Bennett, S.R., F.R. Carbone, F. Karamalis, R.A. Flavell, J.F. Miller, and W.R. Heath. 1998. Help for cytotoxic-T-cell responses is mediated by CD40 signalling [see comments]. *Nature* 393, no. 6684:478.

81. Ridge, J.P., F. Di Rosa, and P. Matzinger. 1998. A conditioned dendritic cell can be a temporal bridge between a CD4+ T- helper and a T-killer cell [see comments]. *Nature* 393, no. 6684:474.

82. Schoenberger, S.P., R.E. Toes, E.I. van der Voort, R. Offringa, and C.J. Melief. 1998. T-cell help for cytotoxic T lymphocytes is mediated by CD40-CD40L interactions [see comments]. *Nature* 393, no. 6684:480.

83. Durie, F.H., A. Aruffo, J. Ledbetter, K.M. Crassi, W.R. Green, L.D. Fast, and R.J. Noelle. 1994. Ab to the ligand of CD40, gp39, blocks the occurrence of the acute and chronic forms of graft-vs-host disease. *J Clin Invest* 94, no. 3:1333.

84. Blazar, B.R., P.A. Taylor, A. Panoskaltsis-Mortari, J. Buhlman, J. Xu, R.A. Flavell, R. Korngold, R. Noelle, and D.A. Vallera. 1997. Blockade of CD40 ligand-CD40 interaction impairs CD4+ T cell-mediated alloreactivity by inhibiting mature donor T cell expansion and function after bone marrow transplantation. *J Immunol* 158, no. 1:29.

85. Buhlmann, J.E., M. Gonzalez, B. Ginther, A. Panoskaltsis-Mortari, B.R. Blazar, D.L. Greiner, A.A. Rossini, R. Flavell, and R.J. Noelle. 1999. Cutting edge: sustained expansion of CD8+ T cells requires CD154 expression by Th cells in acute graft versus host disease. *J Immunol* 162, no. 8:4373.

86. Larsen, C.P., E.T. Elwood, D.Z. Alexander, S.C. Ritchie, R. Hendrix, C. Tucker-Burden, H.R. Cho, A. Aruffo, D. Hollenbaugh, P.S. Linsley, K.J. Winn, and T.C. Pearson. 1996. Long-term acceptance of skin and cardiac allografts after blocking CD40 and CD28 pathways. *Nature* 381, no. 6581:434.

87. Gaspari, A.A., G.D. Sempowski, P. Chess, J. Gish, and R.P. Phipps. 1996. Human epidermal keratinocytes are induced to secrete interleukin-6 and co-stimulate T lymphocyte proliferation by a CD40-dependent mechanism. *Eur J Immunol* 26, no. 6:1371.
88. Hess, S., A. Rensing-Ehl, R. Schwabe, P. Bufler, and H. Engelmann. 1995. CD40 function in nonhematopoietic cells. Nuclear factor kappa B mobilization and induction of IL-6 production. *J Immunol* 155, no. 10:4588.
89. Sempowski, G.D., P.R. Chess, and R.P. Phipps. 1997. CD40 is a functional activation antigen and B7-independent T cell costimulatory molecule on normal human lung fibroblasts. *J Immunol* 158, no. 10:4670.
90. Sempowski, G.D., P.R. Chess, A.J. Moretti, J. Padilla, R.P. Phipps, and T.M. Blieden. 1997. CD40 mediated activation of gingival and periodontal ligament fibroblasts. *J Periodontol* 68, no. 3:284.
91. van Kooten, C., J.S. Gerritsma, M.E. Paape, L.A. van Es, J. Banchereau, and M.R. Daha. 1997. Possible role for CD40-CD40L in the regulation of interstitial infiltration in the kidney. *Kidney Int* 51, no. 3:711.
92. Yellin, M.J., D.A. V, G. Parkinson, A.S. Han, A. Szema, D. Baum, D. Estes, M. Szabolcs, and L. Chess. 1997. Immunohistologic analysis of renal CD40 and CD40L expression in lupus nephritis and other glomerulonephritides. *Arthritis Rheum* 40, no. 1:124.
93. Kalled, S.L., A.H. Cutler, S.K. Datta, and D.W. Thomas. 1998. Anti-CD40 ligand Ab treatment of SNF1 mice with established nephritis: preservation of kidney function. *J Immunol* 160, no. 5:2158.
94. Adawi, A., Y. Zhang, R. Baggs, P. Rubin, J. Williams, J. Finkelstein, and R.P. Phipps. 1998. Blockade of CD40-CD40 ligand interactions protects against radiation- induced pulmonary inflammation and fibrosis. *Clin Immunol Immunopathol* 89, no. 3:222.
95. Adawi, A., Y. Zhang, R. Baggs, J. Finkelstein, and R.P. Phipps. 1998. Disruption of the CD40-CD40 ligand system prevents an oxygen-induced respiratory distress syndrome. *Am J Pathol* 152, no. 3:651.
96. Reul, R.M., J.C. Fang, M.D. Denton, C. Geehan, C. Long, R.N. Mitchell, P. Ganz, and D.M. Briscoe. 1997. CD40 and CD40 ligand (CD154) are coexpressed on microvessels in vivo in human cardiac allograft rejection. *Transplantation* 64, no. 12:1765.
97. Mach, F., U. Schonbeck, G.K. Sukhova, E. Atkinson, and P. Libby. 1998. Reduction of atherosclerosis in mice by inhibition of CD40 signalling. *Nature* 394, no. 6689:200.
98. Schonbeck, U., F. Mach, G.K. Sukhova, E. Atkinson, E. Levesque, M. Herman, P. Graber, P. Basset, and P. Libby. 1999. Expression of stromelysin-3 in atherosclerotic lesions: regulation via CD40-CD40 ligand signaling in vitro and in vivo. *J Exp Med* 189, no. 5:843.
99. Mach, F., U. Schonbeck, R.P. Fabunmi, C. Murphy, E. Atkinson, J.Y. Bonnefoy, P. Graber, and P. Libby. 1999. T lymphocytes induce endothelial cell matrix metalloproteinase expression by a CD40L-dependent mechanism: implications for tubule formation. *Am J Pathol* 154, no. 1:229.
100. Schonbeck, U., F. Mach, G.K. Sukhova, C. Murphy, J.Y. Bonnefoy, R.P. Fabunmi, and P. Libby. 1997. Regulation of matrix metalloproteinase expression in human vascular smooth muscle cells by T lymphocytes: a role for CD40 signaling in plaque rupture? *Circ Res* 81, no. 3:448.
101. Malik, N., B.W. Greenfield, A.F. Wahl, and P.A. Kiener. 1996. Activation of human monocytes through CD40 induces matrix metalloproteinases. *J Immunol* 156, no. 10:3952.
102. Mach, F., U. Schonbeck, R.P. Fabunmi, C. Murphy, E. Atkinson, J.Y. Bonnefoy, P. Graber, and P. Libby. 1999. T lymphocytes induce endothelial cell matrix metalloproteinase expression by a CD40L-dependent mechanism: implications for tubule formation. *Am J Pathol* 154, no. 1:229.
103. Kirk, A.D., L.C. Burkly, D.S. Batty, R.E. Baumgartner, J.D. Berning, K. Buchanan, J.H. Fechner Jr., R.L. Germond, R.L. Kampen, N.B. Patterson, S.J. Swanson, D.K. Tadaki, C.N. Tenhoor, L. White, S.J. Knechtle, and D.M. Harlan. 1999. Treatment with humanized monoclonal Ab against CD154 prevents acute renal allograft rejection in nonhuman primates. *Nature Medicine* 5:686.
104. Kenyon, N.S., M. Chatzipetrou, M. Masetti, A. Ranuncoli, M. Oliveira, J.L. Wagner, A.D. Kirk, D.M. Harlan, L.C. Burkly, and C. Ricordi. 1999. Long-term survival and function of intrahepatic islet allografts in rhesus monkeys treated with humanized anti-CD154. *Proc. Natl. Acad. Sci. USA* 96:8132-8137.
105. Kenyon, N.S., L.A. Fernandez, R. Lehmann, M. Masetti, A. Ranuncoli, M. Chatzipetrou, G. Iaria, D. Han, J.L. Wagner, P. Ruiz, M. Berho, L. Inverardi, R. Alejandro, D.H. Mintz, A.D. Kirk, D.M. Harlan, L.C. Burkly, and C. Ricordi. 1999. Long-term Survival and Function of Intrahepatic islet allografts in baboons treated with humanized anti-CD154. *Diabetes* 48:1473-1481.
106. Mohan, C., Y. Shi, J.D. Laman, and S.K. Datta. 1995. Interaction between CD40 and its ligand gp39 in the development of murine lupus nephritis. *J Immunol* 154, no. 3:1470.

107. Early, G.S., W. Zhao, and C.M. Burns. 1996. Anti-CD40 ligand Ab treatment prevents the development of lupus- like nephritis in a subset of New Zealand black x New Zealand white mice. Response correlates with the absence of an anti-Ab response. *J Immunol* 157, no. 7:3159.
108. Balasa, B., T. Krahl, G. Patstone, J. Lee, R. Tisch, H.O. McDevitt, and N. Sarvetnick. 1997. CD40 ligand-CD40 interactions are necessary for the initiation of insulitis and diabetes in nonobese diabetic mice. *J Immunol* 159, no. 9:4620.
109. Durie, F.H., R.A. Fava, T.M. Foy, A. Aruffo, J.A. Ledbetter, and R.J. Noelle. 1993. Prevention of collagen-induced arthritis with an Ab to gp39, the ligand for CD40. *Science* 261, no. 5126:1328.
110. Gerritse, K., J.D. Laman, R.J. Noelle, A. Aruffo, J.A. Ledbetter, W.J. Boersma, and E. Claassen. 1996. CD40-CD40 ligand interactions in experimental allergic encephalomyelitis and multiple sclerosis. *Proc Natl Acad Sci U S A* 93, no. 6:2499.
111. Howard, L.M., A.J. Miga, C.L. Vanderlugt, M.C. Dal Canto, J.D. Laman, R.J. Noelle, and S.D. Miller. 1999. Mechanisms of immunotherapeutic intervention by anti-CD40L (CD154) Ab in an animal model of multiple sclerosis. *J Clin Invest* 103, no. 2:281.
112. Griggs, N.D., S.S. Agersborg, R.J. Noelle, J.A. Ledbetter, P.S. Linsley, and K.S. Tung. 1996. The relative contribution of the CD28 and gp39 costimulatory pathways in the clonal expansion and pathogenic acquisition of self-reactive T cells. *J Exp Med* 183, no. 3:801.
113. Stuber, E., W. Strober, and M. Neurath. 1996. Blocking the CD40L-CD40 interaction in vivo specifically prevents the priming of T helper 1 cells through the inhibition of interleukin 12 secretion. *J Exp Med* 183, no. 2:693.
114. Seko, Y., N. Takahashi, M. Azuma, H. Yagita, K. Okumura, and Y. Yazaki. 1998. Expression of costimulatory molecule CD40 in murine heart with acute myocarditis and reduction of inflammation by treatment with anti- CD40L/B7-1 monoclonal Abs. *Circ Res* 83, no. 4:463.
115. Larsen, C.P., D.Z. Alexander, D. Hollenbaugh, E.T. Elwood, S.C. Ritchie, A. Aruffo, R. Hendrix, and T.C. Pearson. 1996. CD40-gp39 interactions play a critical role during allograft rejection. Suppression of allograft rejection by blockade of the CD40-gp39 pathway. *Transplantation* 61, no. 1:4.
116. Hancock, W.W., M.H. Sayegh, X.G. Zheng, R. Peach, P.S. Linsley, and L.A. Turka. 1996. Costimulatory function and expression of CD40 ligand, CD80, and CD86 in vascularized murine cardiac allograft rejection. *Proc Natl Acad Sci U S A* 93, no. 24:13967.
117. Lu, L., W. Li, F. Fu, F.G. Chambers, S. Qian, J.J. Fung, and A.W. Thomson. 1997. Blockade of the CD40-CD40 ligand pathway potentiates the capacity of donor-derived dendritic cell progenitors to induce long-term cardiac allograft survival. *Transplantation* 64, no. 12:1808.
118. Niimi, M., T.C. Pearson, C.P. Larsen, D.Z. Alexander, D. Hollenbaugh, A. Aruffo, P.S. Linsley, E. Thomas, K. Campbell, W.C. Fanslow, R.S. Geha, P.J. Morris, and K.J. Wood. 1998. The role of the CD40 pathway in alloantigen-induced hyporesponsiveness in vivo. *J Immunol* 161, no. 10:5331.
119. Fu, F., W. Li, L. Lu, A.W. Thomson, J.J. Fung, and S. Qian. 1999. Systemic administration of CTLA4-Ig or anti-CD40 ligand Ab inhibits second-set rejection of mouse liver allografts. *Transplant Proc* 31, no. 1-2:1244.
120. Sun, H., V. Subbotin, C. Chen, A. Aitouche, L.A. Valdivia, M.H. Sayegh, P.S. Linsley, J.J. Fung, T.E. Starzl, and A.S. Rao. 1997. Prevention of chronic rejection in mouse aortic allografts by combined treatment with CTLA4-Ig and anti-CD40 ligand monoclonal Ab. *Transplantation* 64, no. 12:1838.
121. Markees, T., N. Phillips, E. Gordon, R.J. Noelle, J.P. Mordes, D.L. Greiner, and A.A. Rossini. 1998. Improved skin allograft tolerance induced by treatment with donor splenocytes and an extended course of anti-CD154 monoclonal Ab. *Transplant Proc* 30, no. 5:2444.
122. Markees, T.G., N.E. Phillips, E.J. Gordon, R.J. Noelle, C. Maliszewski, J.P. Mordes, D.L. Greiner, and A.A. Rossini. 1999. Prolonged skin allograft survival in mice treated with Flt3-ligand- induced dendritic cells and anti-CD154 monoclonal Ab. *Transplant Proc* 31, no. 1-2:884.
123. Parker, D.C., D.L. Greiner, N.E. Phillips, M.C. Appel, A.W. Steele, F.H. Durie, R.J. Noelle, J.P. Mordes, and A.A. Rossini. 1995. Survival of mouse pancreatic islet allografts in recipients treated with allogeneic small lymphocytes and Ab to CD40 ligand. *Proc Natl Acad Sci U S A* 92, no. 21:9560.
124. Rossini, A.A., D.C. Parker, N.E. Phillips, F.H. Durie, R.J. Noelle, J.P. Mordes, and D.L. Greiner. 1996. Induction of immunological tolerance to islet allografts. *Cell Transplant* 5, no. 1:49.
125. Rastellini, C., A. Salam, R. Kuddus, A. Aitouche, V. Subbotin, M. Braun, R. Leach, R. Peach, J.J. Fung, T.E. Starzl, and A.S. Rao. 1999. Prevention of T-cell activation by rhCTLA4-Ig and anti-CD40L monoclonal Ab results in indefinite islet allograft survival. *Transplant Proc* 31, no. 1-2:1242.
126. Zheng, X.X., Y. Li, X.C. Li, P. Roy-Chaudhury, P. Nickerson, Y. Tian, M.H. Sayegh, and T.B. Strom. 1999. Blockade of CD40L/CD40 costimulatory pathway in a DST presensitization model of islet allograft leads to a state of Allo-Ag specific tolerance and permits subsequent engraftment of donor strain islet or heart allografts. *Transplant Proc* 31, no. 1-2:627.

127. Gobburu, J.V., C. Tenhoor, M.C. Rogge, D.E. Frazier, Jr., D. Thomas, C. Benjamin, D.M. Hess, and W.J. Jusko. 1998. Pharmacokinetics/dynamics of 5C8, a monoclonal Ab to CD154 (CD40 ligand) suppression of an immune response in monkeys. *J Pharmacol Exp Ther* 286, no. 2:925.
128. Kirk, A.D., D.M. Harlan, N.N. Armstrong, T.A. Davis, Y. Dong, G.S. Gray, X. Hong, D. Thomas, J.H. Fechner, Jr., and S.J. Knechtle. 1997. CTLA4-Ig and anti-CD40 ligand prevent renal allograft rejection in primates. *Proc Natl Acad Sci U S A* 94, no. 16:8789.
129. Chang, A.C., M.G. Blum, K.S. Blair, M.A. Scott, J.E. Brock, D.W. Thomas, L.C. Burkly, G.G. Miller, and R.N. Pierson, 3rd. 1999. Prolonged anti-CD40 ligand therapy improves primate cardiac allograft survival. *Transplant Proc* 31, no. 1-2:95.
130. Bachmann, M.F., R.M. Zinkernagel, and A. Oxenius. 1998. Immune responses in the absence of costimulation: viruses know the trick. *J Immunol* 161, no. 11:5791.
131. Whitmire, J.K., M.K. Slifka, I.S. Grewal, R.A. Flavell, and R. Ahmed. 1996. CD40 ligand-deficient mice generate a normal primary cytotoxic T- lymphocyte response but a defective humoral response to a viral infection [published erratum appears in J Virol 1997 Feb;71(2):1736]. *J Virol* 70, no. 12:8375.
132. Oxenius, A., K.A. Campbell, C.R. Maliszewski, T. Kishimoto, H. Kikutani, H. Hengartner, R.M. Zinkernagel, and M.F. Bachmann. 1996. CD40-CD40 ligand interactions are critical in T-B cooperation but not for other anti-viral CD4+ T cell functions. *J Exp Med* 183, no. 5:2209.
133. Borrow, P., A. Tishon, S. Lee, J. Xu, I.S. Grewal, M.B. Oldstone, and R.A. Flavell. 1996. CD40L-deficient mice show deficits in antiviral immunity and have an impaired memory CD8+ CTL response. *J Exp Med* 183, no. 5:2129.
134. Borrow, P., D.F. Tough, D. Eto, A. Tishon, I.S. Grewal, J. Sprent, R.A. Flavell, and M.B. Oldstone. 1998. CD40 ligand-mediated interactions are involved in the generation of memory CD8(+) cytotoxic T lymphocytes (CTL) but are not required for the maintenance of CTL memory following virus infection. *J Virol* 72, no. 9:7440.
135. Anderson, D.M., E. Maraskovsky, W.L. Billingsley, W.C. Dougall, M.E. Tometsko, E.R. Roux, M.C. Teepe, R.F. DuBose, D. Cosman, and L. Galibert. 1997. A homologue of the TNF receptor and its ligand enhance T-cell growth and dendritic-cell function. *Nature* 390, no. 6656:175.
136. Wong, B.R., R. Josien, S.Y. Lee, B. Sauter, H.L. Li, R.M. Steinman, and Y. Choi. 1997. TRANCE (tumor necrosis factor [TNF]-related activation-induced cytokine), a new TNF family member predominantly expressed in T cells, is a dendritic cell-specific survival factor. *J Exp Med* 186, no. 12:2075.
137. Wong, B.R., J. Rho, J. Arron, E. Robinson, J. Orlinick, M. Chao, S. Kalachikov, E. Cayani, F.S. Bartlett, 3rd, W.N. Frankel, S.Y. Lee, and Y. Choi. 1997. TRANCE is a novel ligand of the tumor necrosis factor receptor family that activates c-Jun N-terminal kinase in T cells. *J Biol Chem* 272, no. 40:25190.
138. Green, E.A., and R.A. Flavell. 1999. TRANCE-RANK, a new signal pathway involved in lymphocyte development and T cell activation [comment]. *J Exp Med* 189, no. 7:1017.
139. Bachmann, M.F., B.R. Wong, R. Josien, R.M. Steinman, A. Oxenius, and Y. Choi. 1999. TRANCE, a tumor necrosis factor family member critical for CD40 ligand- independent T helper cell activation [see comments]. *J Exp Med* 189, no. 7:1025.
140. Yang, Y., Q. Su, I.S. Grewal, R. Schilz, R.A. Flavell, and J.M. Wilson. 1996. Transient subversion of CD40 ligand function diminishes immune responses to adenovirus vectors in mouse liver and lung tissues. *J Virol* 70, no. 9:6370.
141. Yang, Y., and J.M. Wilson. 1996. CD40 ligand-dependent T cell activation: requirement of B7-CD28 signaling through CD40. *Science* 273, no. 5283:1862.
142. Wilson, C.B., L.J. Embree, D. Schowalter, R. Albert, A. Aruffo, D. Hollenbaugh, P. Linsley, and M.A. Kay. 1998. Transient inhibition of CD28 and CD40 ligand interactions prolongs adenovirus-mediated transgene expression in the lung and facilitates expression after secondary vector administration. *J Virol* 72, no. 9:7542.
143. Scaria, A., J.A. St George, R.J. Gregory, R.J. Noelle, S.C. Wadsworth, A.E. Smith, and J.M. Kaplan. 1997. Ab to CD40 ligand inhibits both humoral and cellular immune responses to adenoviral vectors and facilitates repeated administration to mouse airway. *Gene Ther* 4, no. 6:611.
144. Kay, M.A., L. Meuse, A.M. Gown, P. Linsley, D. Hollenbaugh, A. Aruffo, H.D. Ochs, and C.B. Wilson. 1997. Transient immunomodulation with anti-CD40 ligand Ab and CTLA4Ig enhances persistence and secondary adenovirus-mediated gene transfer into mouse liver. *Proc Natl Acad Sci U S A* 94, no. 9:4686.

1. THE TREATMENT OF BLEEDING EPISODES IN PATIENTS WITH FACTOR VIII INHIBITORS: A DATA SYNTHESIS

Martin L. Lee*, PhD,Werner Urbancik, Ph.D, Gordon Bray, MD., Edward Gomperts, MD.
University of California, Los Angeles and Baxter Healthcare Corporation, Vienna, Austria and Glendale, California, USA

Factor VIII bypassing agents have been employed since the early 1970's as a means of treating hemophilia patients with inhibitors (alloantibodies) to Factor VIII or Factor IX. There is a large body of published work in this regard, but the vast majority is anecdotal, consisting of single case reports or small patient series. There are, however, several randomized, controlled trials. We chose to summarize this information along with the open-label results in order to provide an overall picture of the safety and efficacy of these agents in this clinical setting. We used both the controlled and uncontrolled data in this synthesis, since the latter provide an interesting contrast to the former insofar as the positive observer bias in results seen, as well as providing a larger database for evaluating and comparing these preparations. We focused on hemarthroses, since this type of bleeding episode tends to be more comparable across patients and studies. (cf. Lusher et al, 1980). Four different types of preparations were evaluated: rVIIa (NovoSeven), activated prothrombin complex concentrates (aPCC): FEIBA and Autoplex, and Factor IX complex (PCC). The results from the prospective controlled trials show a remarkably narrow range of effectiveness (adjusting for the different study metrics) of 50-78% with the Factor IX Complexes yielding the numerically lowest findings. However, the number of doses of study product appeared to be higher for rVIIa compared to the plasma-based preparations, where a single dose usually sufficed. Interestingly, rates of response to two infusions of NovoSeven (cf. Keyes 1998) approximate those observed in association with one infusion of placebo in the randomized prospective controlled studies of PCCs (cf. Lusher, 1980). Interestingly, all products performed much better (>80% effectiveness) in open trials (versus randomized studies) and by an amount roughly equal to the aforementioned placebo effect (or 25%). All preparations had a relatively similar acute adverse event profile. We conclude that there is little evidence to support superior hemostatic efficacy of one product category versus any other in the management of hemarthroses but the lower dose frequency may favor aPCCs. This data synthesis also emphasizes the importance of randomized, prospective controlled studies in the evaluation of bypassing agents as there is a clear and quantifiable placebo effect.

2. THREE CASES OF ACQUIRED VON WILLEBRAND DISEASE ASSOCIATED WITH SYSTEMIC LUPUS ERYTHEMATOSUS.

Paquita Nurden[*1] Jean-Luc Pellegrin[2], Christine Vergnes[1], Annie Borel-Derlon[3], Gisèle Clofent-Sanchez[2], Bernard Leng[2], Jean-François Viallard[2], Alan T. Nurden[1]. UMR 5533 CNRS, Hôpital Cardiologique,[1] Clinique de Médecine Interne et Maladies Infectieuses, Hôpital Haut-Lévêque,[2] Pessac, Laboratoire d'Hématologie, CHU de Caen,[3] France.

Although von Willebrand disease (vWD) is among the most common of the congenital haemorrhagic syndromes, acquired forms have only rarely been reported. Acquired vWD is usually associated with autoimmune or clonal proliferative disorders suggesting an immunologic origin. We now report three cases of acquired vWD associated with systemic lupus erythematosus (SLE) that have been detected in three middle-aged women. In each case, the first clinical manifestation of the disease was a bleeding syndrome and SLE was diagnosed subsequently.

Patient 1 with the mildest clinical manifestation resembled type 1 vWD and has 20% vWF:RCo, 23% vWF:Ag and 42% FVIII:C. The second patient can be compared to type 3 since vWF:RCo was < 1%, while 4% vWF:Ag and 8% FVIII:C were present, although a case could also be made for a severe type 1 deficiency. Finally, patient 3 possessed 13% vWF:RCo activity but 94% vWF:Ag and 76% VIII:C. Ristocetin-induced agglutination of the patient's platelets was much reduced, and the high molecular weight vWF multimers were decreased following their analysis by electrophoresis, thereby suggesting type 2 vWD. Patient 3 also showed a moderate anaemia and a platelet count >900,000/μL. For each patient, mixing patient's plasma with normal plasma resulted in inhibition of the agglutination of control platelets in the presence of ristocetin. For patients 1 and 2, IgG, IgM and IgA antibodies were detected when using purified vWF in a fluorescence-based microplate assay. For patient 3, only IgG antibodies were present, as has been reported for the majority of cases of acquired vWD. Significantly, intraplatelet levels of vWF were normal for all three patients. The three cases that we report here illustrate the difficulty in characterizing acquired vWD, which may have a variable phenotype.

For patient 1, with moderate clinical signs, and quiescent SLE, no treatment was started. In contrast, IVIgG were given to patients 2 and 3, but benefit was only observed for patient 2 and this was not sustained beyond 15 to 20 days. It is interesting to note for this patient that after IVIgG infusion, not only vWF but also FVIII:C levels increased, whereas after transfusion of purified vWF no modifications were observed in FVIII:C levels. This is probably due to the fact that transfusion of purified vWF for this patient was only followed by a short duration (30 min) increase in vWF, implying that a powerful inhibitor was present in the circulation. Probably the transfused vWF did not remain a sufficient time in the circulation to protect against the effect of the inhibitor. Also for patient 2, the appearance of severe nonscarring papulosquamous lesions was treated by corticosteroids. But an aggravation of the lesions led us to start cyclophosphamide treatment. With this latter therapy, a total correction of the vWF levels was obtained. For patient 3, increased vWF levels and correction of blood parameters were seen after corticosteroid treatment, but not following IVIgG infusion. These three cases illustrate the heterogeneity in the response to treatment.

Of considerable interest was the fact that each patient mimicked a different congenital form of vWD. Furthermore, these cases underline the necessity to look for an acquired form of vWD when decreased vWF levels are detected without a family history of bleeding and evidence for a congenital defect. Such observations also highlight the necessity to look for autoimmune disease when a decreased vWF level is found in adults and where the disease may in fact be acquired.

3. FACTOR IX DENVER: ASN 346_ ASP MUTATION RESULTING IN A DYSFUNCTIONAL PROTEIN WITH A DECREASED AFFINITY FOR FACTOR VIIIA.

J.B. Lefkowitz*, R. Nuss, A. Thompson, T. Haver, L. Jacobson, and M. Manco-Johnson._ Departments of Pathology and Pediatrics, University of Colorado Health Sciences Center, Denver, CO and Puget Sound Blood Center, Seattle WA.

An obligate carrier of mild hemophilia B presented with severe right groin pain with no history of preceding trauma. CT scanning confirmed hemorrhage in the iliacus muscle causing objective signs of nerve compression. After failing conservative therapy she was treated with factor IX concentrate . She improved symptomatically but ultimately developed a pseudotumor. Her father had a history of more severe bleeding than would be expected from his assayed factor IX (FIX) level. Because of these findings this family was studied in detail, as shown:

Subject	FIX Activity U/dL	FIX Antigen U/dL
Proband male	26	170
Carrier daughter	67	165
Affected son of carrier	21	118

Sequencing of genomic DNA of these three family members revealed a single base transition in codon 346 (AAC_ GAC) in the 8th exon of the FIX gene which predicts an amino acid change of Asn 346_ Asp. The female was heterozygous for this mutation. The proband male was plasmapheresed and approximately 400 mL of citrated plasma was removed for purification of FIX Denver. FIX Denver was purified using ion exchange and immunoaffinity chromatography. The isolated protein was >99% pure on a silver stained SDS-PAGE and had a specific activity of 22.5 U/mg compared with purified native FIX of 309 U/mg. Clotting assays using FIX deficient plasma reconstituted with purified native or Denver FIX showed results similar to that of the whole starting plasmas. Phospholipid vesicles (PL: 27% phosphatidylserine , 73% phosphatidyl- choline) were made by extrusion. PL in concentrations from 1 to 2000 _M showed similar interactions with equimolar concentrations of native or Denver FIX in the activation of factor X using Spectrozyme FXa as a chromogen. Kinetic constants for interactions of FIXa with factor X/PL and factor X/PL/factor VIIIa were performed using a kinetic plate reader and Spectrozyme FXa. Factor X interactions with native and Denver factor IXa/PL showed a Km of 253 vs 263 nM; Vmax of 0.056 vs 0.041 nM FXa/min. Factor X interaction with native or Denver FIXa/PL/factor VIIIa showed a Km of 57.5 vs. 57.1 nM; Vmax of 5.58 vs. 1.69 nM factor Xa/min. The Kd of FIXa Denver for factor VIIIa is 9.85 nM while the Kd of FIXa native for FVIIIa is 0.095 nM. The major defect caused by this point mutation is a marked decrease in the affinity of FIXa Denver for FVIIIa. Adapted with permission from Blood 92: abstract 756, p. 187a, 1998.

4. CARDIAC SURGERY COMPLICATED BY HEPARIN REBOUND IN A PATIENT WITH F.XI INHIBITOR ASSOCIATED WITH CONGENITAL F.XI DEFICIENCY Jun Teruya* and Michael Styler, Hahnemann University Hospital, Philadelphia, PA

Case: A 77-year old Caucasian male of Jewish extraction was scheduled for cardiac surgery to repair aortic stenosis. His past medical history is remarkable for tonsillectomy, inguinal hernia repair, elbow surgery, bilateral total knee replacement, hemorrhoidectomy, and aortocoronary bypass 3 years before. When he underwent hernia surgery, he required 3 units of packed red cell transfusion. He was then diagnosed as having F.XI deficiency. He was found to have an inhibitor to F.XI 3 years ago.
Lab data: PTT 81.9 sec, PTT mixing study; 42.4 sec at 0 min and 54.4 sec after 2-hour incubation (normal PTT 24.4 sec to 35.5 sec), F.XI level 1%, dilute Russell's viper venom test negative, F.XI inhibitor titer; 1.6 BU.
Hospital course: Plasmapheresis was performed before cardiac catheterization using a dual lumen catheter inserted through the right femoral vein. A 1.5 plasma volume exchange was completed using 5% albumin for the first half and fresh frozen plasma (FFP) for the second half. The PTT was shortened to 37.3 seconds from 81.9 seconds and the F.XI level was increased to 22% from 1%. A 1:1 mixing study of PTT after the plasmapheresis showed complete correction into the normal range, which suggests no inhibitor was present. When he went to cardiac surgery, PTT was 31.6 sec, PT was 14.8 sec, and TT was 15.4 sec after another plasmapheresis. Cardiac surgery was uneventful and the PTT was 44.5 sec after protamine was given. Six hours after surgery, he started to bleed from the chest tubes. The PTT was 111.3 sec, PT was 16.1 sec, and TT was 120.0 sec at that time. After additional 50 mg of protamine was given, bleeding stopped and the PTT and TT were shortened to 36.1 sec and 13.8 sec, respectively. Four days after surgery another 1.5 plasma volume exchange was performed because the patient was going to have the cardiac pacing wire removed. However, the PTT was shortened to only 78.5 sec from 93.6 sec. On the following day a same volume exchange was performed without any effect on PTT: 74.4 sec and 75.7 sec, before and after plasmapheresis, respectively. The F.XI level was found to be <1%. The cardiac pacing wire was then cut under the skin instead of taking out from the heart muscle due to the prolonged PTT. Although the patient later developed a subileus, he was discharged without further complications.
Discussion: Among homozygous F.XI deficiency, 50% individuals are bleeders and 50% are non-bleeders. This patient has homozygous F.XI deficiency and was found to be a bleeder due to his significant past bleeding history after surgery. For repeated transfusion of FFP, he acquired a F.XI inhibitor. He received a total of 7 plasmapheresis procedures over 8 days. While albumin was used for the first 2 procedures to minimize the antibody stimulation, the 6th and 7th plasmaphereses were of no effect to remove the F.XI inhibitor and increase F.XI level. Although it was thought to be due to elevation of the inhibitor titer, an inhibitor assay analogous to F.VIII inhibitor assay demonstrated 1.6 BU, which was the same as his baseline level.

Heparin rebound occurs between 1 and 9 hours after surgery. Since this patient did not receive heparin after surgery, there was no ongoing source of heparin. His prolonged PTT and TT with a normal PT were corrected by protamine administration. This evidence strongly suggests that the patient had heparin rebound. While the incidence of heparin rebound is reported up to 50% of patients after cardiac surgery, most cases are unrecognized without causing major bleeding.

5. CANINE HEMOPHILIA: A NATURALLY OCCURRING AND HETEROGENEOUS ANIMAL MODEL

*Marjory B. Brooks[1], Kunal Ray[2], Weikuan Gu[2], James Catalfamo[1], Jharna Ray[2]
[1] Comparative Coagulation Section, Dept. Population Medicine & Diagnostic Science, and
[2] James Baker Institute for Animal Health, College of Vet. Med., Cornell University, Ithaca, NY

Canine hemophilia is an established animal model of the human disease. The molecular basis of canine hemophilia B is known for two research colonies, each derived from a single founder male. Hemophilia, however, occurs frequently as a naturally occurring coagulopathy in companion animal dogs. Through the Coagulation Section's diagnostic program, cases of hemophilia A and B are routinely identified in many different purebred and mixed-breed dogs. Clinical features of canine hemophilia parallel the human disease. The incidence of canine hemophilia A is approximately 4 to 5 times that of hemophilia B and both defects are phenotypically heterogeneous. Mild, moderate, and severe forms occur, with *in vitro* factor VIII and IX coagulant activity predictive of clinical severity. Each canine breed represents a closed breeding population. On the basis of pedigree review and familial testing, cases of canine hemophilia appear to arise from familial transmission and from new mutations. Analogous to human populations, founder effect is most important in propagation of mild hemophilia.

In preliminary analyses of canine hemophilia B, we found that molecular heterogeneity underlies observed phenotypic variability. Ten distinct breed-variants were studied, including mild, moderate, and severe disease phenotypes. Southern blot analyses, using a full-length canine factor IX cDNA probe, revealed variant hybridization patterns for 5 dogs. Using primers to specifically amplify each of the 8 canine factor IX exons, we further defined mutations in 3 of these dogs. Using primers to amplify across exons, we identified a mutation in a fourth dog. Three mutations caused severe hemophilia, including a complete factor IX gene deletion, a partial gene deletion spanning exons 1 to 6, and a 5 kb insertion in exon 8 that caused aberrant splicing and truncation of the factor IX transcript. The fourth mutation consisted of a 1.3 kb insertion in intron 5, and was associated with a mild hemophilia phenotype (fIX:C = 10%). Both large gene insertions were flanked by direct repeats, suggestive of retrotransposition of LINE 1 elements as the mutation mechanism. We are continuing to characterize the canine factor IX gene, by determining intron organization and sequence of each splice junction in order to detect missense and small insertion/deletion mutations in genomic DNA of affected males.

Canine models have been successfully utilized for *in vivo* efficacy and toxicity studies of plasma-derived and recombinant factor concentrates. New applications for a large animal model of hemophilia include development of somatic cell gene therapy and strategies to ameliorate or prevent inhibitor formation. The potential for testing novel strategies in dogs having different mutations enhances the model's value for predicting response in mutationally heterogeneous human populations. Comparative studies of factor VIII and IX mutations will also provide insight into spontaneous mutation mechanisms on the X chromosome of mammalian species.

6. DOES AGE AT FIRST TREATMENT INFLUENCE FVIII INHIBITOR LEVELS?

DL Aronson*1, Gordon Bray2, David Ramies3, Chantal Rothschild4, Evan Vosburgh2. 1. Unaffiliated, 2 Baxter-Immuno, 3.Bayer, 4 Hopital Necker

Inhibitors remain a major problem in the treatment of hemophilia A. As many as 30% of previously untreated patients (PUP) have a measurable inhibitor at some time. Risk factors for inhibitors have been shown to be for the most part genetically determined. Patients with an intron 22 inversion, large deletions and nonsense mutations are at higher risk than other hemophilia A genotypes for developing an inhibitor. In addition, product(rarely) and race have been associated with the development of inhibitors.

Variables impacting on the inhibitor titers have not been examined. Tolerance to antigens can be acquired in-utero but also during the peri-natal period. If so, lower inhibitor levels might be seen with earlier treatment of patients with hemophilia..

Data from 3 recombinant Factor VIII PUP trials, with a total of 170 patients, which includes 57 patients with inhibitors, have been compiled (1-3). These have been analyzed for any relationship between the age of first treatment and the maximum inhibitor levels observed.

The first treatment for inhibitor patients was at a median age of 8 months and an average of 6.5 months; non-inhibitor patients were treated at a median age of 10 months and a mean of 12.4 months. Sixteen patients without inhibitors had their first treatment at more than 28 months and probably represents less severe patients at lower risk of inhibitor formation. All patients who developed an inhibitor were first treated before 25 months of age.This difference was not significant.

The median peak inhibitor titer for patients treated before 9 months was 5.8 Bethesda Units and for those treated at or after 9 months was 8.9 Bethesda Units. There is no significant difference between inhibitor titers before and after 9 months. The tests applied were (2 comparing patients with inhibitor titers of less than 20 u/mL and 20 or greater u/mL and Mann-Whitney U test to test the relationship of inhibitor titer and age as a continuous variable.

References

1. Lusher JM, Arkin S, Abilgaard CF, Hurst D. Recombinant factor VIII(Kogenate) treatment of previously untreated patients(PUPS) with hemophilia A: Update of safety, efficacy and inhibitor development after seven study years.Thromb Haemostas 1997;78 (supplement): Abstract PD-664.

2. Gruppo R, Chen H, Schroth P et al. Safety and immunogenicity of recombinant Factor VIII (Recombinate) in previously untreated patients (PUPS). A 7.5 year update. Haemophilia 1998; Abstract #291.
3. Rothschild C, Laurian Y, Satre EP, et al. French Previously untreated patients with severe hemophilia A after exposure to recombinant factor VIII: Incidence of inhibitor and evaluation of immune tolerance. Thromb Haemost 1998;80:779-83.

7. ANTI-FACTOR VIII (FVIII) HUMAN MONOCLONAL ANTIBODIES WITH COMPLEX KINETICS OF FVIII INACTIVATION.

M. Jacquemin, J.G. Gilles*, B. Desqueper, R. Lavend'homme, K. Peerlinck, J. Vermylen, and J.M.R. Saint-Remy. Center for Molecular and Vascular Biology, University of Leuven, Leuven, Belgium.

Seven to 25% of hemophilia A patients produce antibodies directed towards FVIII in response to FVIII concentrate infusion. Those antibodies, called inhibitors, are detected by their ability to interfere with FVIII activity in coagulation or chromogenic assays. However, both the detection and quantification of FVIII inhibitor remain difficult, notably, because different types of FVIII inhibitor can be distinguished according to the pattern of FVIII inactivation.

Biggs et al. distinguished antibodies inactivating FVIII following a pseudo-first order kinetics and antibodies with a more complex pattern of FVIII inactivation, with which FVIII inactivation was very often incomplete (1). Antibodies inactivating FVIII completely following a pseudo-first order kinetics were then called Type I inhibitor, whereas antibodies which inactivate FVIII incompletely following a complex kinetics were called Type II inhibitors (2).

The mechanism of action of antibodies with complex pattern of FVIII inactivation remains poorly understood and proved difficult to analyse with patient polyclonal antibodies. We therefore analysed two human monoclonal antibodies exhibiting complex kinetics of FVIII inactivation. Both antibodies were obtained by immortalisation of peripheral blood lymphocytes of hemophilia A patients with inhibitor (3, 4).

The first antibody, BO2C11, recognises the FVIII C2 domain and inhibits FVIII binding to phosphatidylserine. B02C11 also inhibits FVIII binding to vWF. Conversely, the rate of inactivation of FVIII by BO2C11 is reduced in the presence of vWF, much alike what was described with Type II polyclonal antibodies (2). However, in the presence of an excess of B02C11, and after prolonged incubation time periods, FVIII inactivation is complete, due to the fact that the affinity of BO2C11 for FVIII is 10-fold higher than that of vWF. This antibody therefore does not match the definition of either a type I or a type II inhibitor, but yet corresponds to a frequently encountered population of inhibitors able to completely inactivate FVIII, albeit with complex kinetics (5).

The second antibody, LE2E9 recognises the FVIII C1 domain. Used in large excess over vWF, LE2E9 inactivates only 85% of FVIII activity in plasma, like a typical type II inhibitor. However, LE2E9 inhibits only 85% of purified rFVIII. Therefore, LE2E9 represents a novel variant of type II inhibitor, which mechanism of FVIII inactivation is independent of the presence of vWF.

The characterisation of FVIII inactivation by these two human monoclonal antibodies, BO2C11 and LE2E9, illustrates the diversity of FVIII inhibitors with complex kinetics of FVIII inactivation, which is likely to contribute to the difficulties inherent to the standardization of FVIII inhibitor assays.

1. Biggs R. et al.The mode of action of antibodies which destroy factor VIII. II. Antibodies which give complex concentration graphs. British J. Haematol. 1972, 23:137.
2. Gawryl M. et al. Inactivation of factor VIII coagulant activity by two different types of human antibodies. Blood 1982, 60:1103.
3. Jacquemin M. et al. Mechanism and kinetics of factor VIII inactivation: study with an IgG4 monoclonal antibody derived from a hemophilia A patient with inhibitor. Blood 1998, 92:496.
4. Peerlinck K. et al.. Antifactor VIII antibody inhibiting allogeneic but not autologous factor VIII in patients with mild hemophilia A. Blood in press
5. Biggs R. Antibodies to factor VIII clotting activity (VIII:C). In: Human Blood Coagulation, Haemostasis and Thrombosis (third edition). Biggs R, Rizza CR, eds Blackwell Scientific Publications, Oxford 1984; pp205.

8. THE HEMOPHILIA RESEARCH SOCIETY OF NORTH AMERICA(HRS)/NOVO NORDISK HEMOPHILIA REGISTRY.

Craig M. Kessler* and Joan C. Gill, Georgetown University Medical Center, Washington, DC; and Comprehensive Center for Bleeding Disorders, Milwaukee, WI

The HRS/Novo Nordisk Hemophilia Registry is a unique collaboration between industry and the academic medical community caring for individuals with hemophilia. This patient tracking system is designed to serve as a national database and monitoring device intended to analyze the efficacy and safety of NovoSeven in the market place. Treatment trends, patient and physician choice of products for therapy, and complications associated with the various therapies will be tracked for all allo and autoantibody inhibitor patients. Of primary importance is the fact that this Hemophilia Registry provides an efficient mechanism via a computer network available to all hemophilia treatment centers (HTCs) whereby adverse events associated with administration of NovoSeven and other concentrates to inhibitor patients can be reported rapidly to the Food and Drug Administration (FDA). In addition, the format of the Hemophilia Registry will facilitate integration of patient information into the longitudinal database coordinated by the Centers for Disease Control and Prevention (CDCP) for federally funded HTCs. This patient tracking system offers several important advantages: 1) It has enhanced reporting capabilities and offers the NHRR bulletin board to discuss/pose clinical or research questions with other hematologists authorized to utilize the network; 2) It is user friendly with features like electronic submission of data, online help and a toll-free helpline to answer any questions; 3) The confidentiality of patients will be safeguarded by introducing sophisticated encryption codes and patient identifiers; and 4) It will enhance quality control and data accuracy by real-time data cleaning and linked forms. The contents of the database will be owned by the HRS and be made available to their membership for academic activities and generation of publications. The HRS/Novo Nordisk Hemophilia Registry and NovoSeven patient tracking system will allow HTCs to understand the characteristics of patients with hemophilia and inhibitors and to observe treatment trends and outcomes.

9. SAFETY AND EFFICACY OF COAGULATION FACTOR VIIa (RECOMBINANT) WHEN ADMINISTERED AS I.V. BOLUS OR I.V. CONTINUOUS INFUSION TO HEMOPHILIA A OR B PATIENTS WITH INHIBITORS UNDERGOING ELECTIVE MAJOR SURGICAL PROCEDURES.

G. S. Gilchrist*, D. Green, K. Hoots, B. A. Konkle, and E. Erhardtsen, Hemophilia Center, Mayo Clinic, Rochester MN; Northwestern University, Chicago, IL; University of Texas Science Center, Houston, TX; Thomas Jefferson University, Philadelphia, PA; Novo Nordisk Pharmaceuticals, Inc., Princeton, NJ.

Treatment of patients with hemophilia and inhibitors or acquired inhibitors against Factor VIII or IX represent a major challenge to clinicians. Activated recombinant coagulation factor VII (rFVIIa) is a newly developed approach to the treatment of these patients. An ongoing open-label, randomized trial in the US is comparing safety and efficacy of rFVIIa administered by continuous infusion or by bolus injection to patients with inhibitors undergoing elective major surgical procedures. In the continuous infusion group, rFVIIa is administered as an intravenous bolus injection of 90μg/kg just prior to surgery followed by continuous infusion at 50μg/kg/hr for the first five days of treatment and then at no less than one-half the rate from day 6 to day 10. In the bolus dosing group, rFVIIa is administered at 90μg/kg by i.v. injection just prior to surgery. Dosing is continued at least every 2 hours or as required during surgery until wound closure and then continued at 2 hour intervals for the first five days and then at 4 hour intervals from day 6 to day 10. A third, non-randomized, non-inhibitor hemophiliac A or B patient group undergoing similar surgery and treatment with FVIII or FIX for hemostasis is being studied as a control group. Efficacy is assessed by evaluating the achievement and maintenance of hemostasis during and after surgery. The levels of clotting activity of factor seven (FVII:C) are measured at different time points to correlate with the hemostatic effect. Patients are monitored for the adverse events and laboratory abnormalities. As of 2/15/99 five patients have been studied, three patients (eye surgery; abdominal psuedotumor; cholecystectomy) by IV bolus and two patients (partial resection of brain tumor; synovectomy) by continuous infusion.

10. PHARMACOKINETICS OF RECOMBINANT ACTIVATED FACTOR VII (rFVIIa).

E. Erhardtsen*, Novo Nordisk Pharmaceuticals, Inc., Princeton, NJ

Recombinant activated factor VII (rFVIIa) is being used to control bleeding in patients with hemophilia and is reported to be safe and effective in normalizing prothrombin time (PT) in patients with cirrhosis and in healthy volunteers pre-treated with the oral anticoagulant acenocoumarol. The pharmacokinetics of rFVIIa have been evaluated in adult patients with hemophilia A or B, adult patients with cirrhosis and a prolonged PT, and healthy adult volunteers who were pre-treated with acenocoumarol. The clearance and half-life of rFVIIa were similar in the adult populations studied: patients with hemophilia, patients with cirrhosis, and healthy volunteers. The volume of distribution at steady state (V_{SS}) on the other hand, was slightly smaller in healthy adult volunteers (who were pre-treated with acenocoumarol) as compared to patients with hemophilia (not calculated for adult patients with cirrhosis and prolonged PT). The pharmacokinetic profile of rFVIIa seems to be independent of bleeding or non-bleeding conditions in adult hemophilia patients; only slightly shorter half-life (2.48 vs. 2.82 hours) and increased clearance values (36.6 vs. 32.1 ml/kg/hr) were observed in the bleeding episodes as compared to the non-bleeding episodes. However, it must be emphasized that the patients in these studies did not suffer from major bleeding episodes. The pharmacokinetic parameters (clearance and half-life) were also dose-independent in adult patients with hemophilia and in the patients with cirrhosis (dose dependency not determined in healthy volunteers).

Pharmacokinetic Parameters	Adult patients with hemophilia A or B (n=15)	Adult patients with cirrhosis (n=10)	Adult healthy volunteers (n=28)
$t_{1/2}$ (hours)	2.72± 0.54	2.87	2.45±0.25
CL (ml/kg/hr)	32.8±11.7	34.9±16.5	34.5±7.0
Vss (ml/kg)	108.9±37.2	Not calculated	93.6±14.5

11. SUBCUTANEOUS RECOMBINANT HUMAN FACTOR IX (BeneFix™) REDUCES HEMORRHAGIC EPISODES IN TOLERIZEED HEMOPHILIA B DOGS OVER ONE YEAR

KE Russell[1], TC Nichols[1], RL Mustafa[1], DA Bellinger[1], BJ Rup[2], KP McCarthy[2], RG Schaub[2], MS Read[1] Department of Pathology and Laboratory Medicine, UNC, Chapel Hill, NC[1] and Genetics Institute, Inc., Andover, MA[2]

Hemorrhagic events in the Chapel Hill strain of hemophilia B dogs are frequent, severe, and fatal if not treated promptly. Currently, replacement therapy with normal canine plasma is given to treat hemorrhagic events. We hypothesized that the incidence of bleeding episodes could be reduced by sustained prophylactic treatment. To test this hypothesis, hemophilia B dogs tolerant to recombinant human factor IX (rF.IX) (Blood 1998 92:2280a) were given rF.IX subcutaneously (SC) for 14 months. rF.IX was administered SC, a relatively easy and feasible approach (Throm Haemost 1997 77:944). The whole blood clotting time (WBCT), APTT, and incidence of hemorrhagic episodes were determined and compared to hemophilia B dogs that formed Bethesda inhibitors (BIU) to rF.IX and wild-type hemophilia B dogs in the colony. The WBCT and APTT in normal dogs in the Chapel Hill colony is 8-12 minutes and 28-32 seconds, respectively. In untreated hemophilia B dogs, WBCT is >50 minutes and APTT is 80-108 seconds.

Table 1 WBCT (minutes)

	Day	88	107	240	268	303	331	359	401
Tolerized[1]	C20	16.5	12.5	12.5	12.5	13.5	12.5	11.5	11.5
	C22	15.5	10	11.5	12.5	12.5	11.5	11.5	11.5
	C23	21	11	12	12	12.5	12	12.5	12.5
	C25	16	11.5	14	12	13	12	11.5	12.5
	C26	17	12	12.5	13	13.5	13	12.5	13.5
Inhibitor[1,2]	C19	>60	24.5						
	C24	>60	>60						
	C27	>60	>60						

Table 2 APTT (seconds)

	Day	88	107	240	268	303	331	359	401
Tolerized[1]	C20	84.8	73.7	64.7	76.4	65.9	59.3	75.1	56.5
	C22	81.2	67.8	70.4	72.2	77.9	72.1	70.7	75.7
	C23	93.1	68.3	63.5	68.8	68.9	79.4	78.2	63.9
	C25	77.3	62.2	64.2	73.8	81.8	65.5	67.4	79.3
	C26	92.1	77.1	71.6	88.4	75.5	62.6	70.2	60.4
Inhibitor[1,2]	C19	100.7	91.8						
	C24	101	103.9						
	C27	104.6	114.3						

[1] Tolerized dogs had no detectable Bethesda inhibitors; inhibitor dogs developed 3, 0.9, and 6 BIU, respectively.
[2] Dogs were removed from study on day 107 due to inhibitor formation

Table 3 Average Number of Hemorrhagic Episodes/Dog/Year in Hemophilia B Dogs

	Number of dogs	Hemorrhagic Episodes
Tolerized Dogs	5	1.60
Inhibitor Dogs	3	7.55
Wild-type Hemophilia B Dogs	40	5.78

During treatment with rF.IX, the tolerized dogs exhibited shortened WBCT and APTT compared to the inhibitor dogs and wild-type hemophilia B dogs (Tables 1, 2). The tolerized dogs had a reduction in bleeding episodes with twice weekly SC dosing of rF.IX (Table 3). These data justify the consideration of prophylactic treatment of human hemophilia B patients with SC rF.IX to reduce bleeding episodes.

12. CHARACTERIZATION OF FACTOR IX INHIBITOR ANTIBODIES

K.Charleston, J.Heimbaugh, M.Switzer, K. Leitermann, B.Rup*.
Genetics Institute, Andover, MA

Although development of antibodies that inhibit clotting activity of Factor IX (FIX) is rare in hemophilia B patients, presence of such antibodies (inhibitors) represents a serious complication of FIX replacement therapy. Inhibitor antibodies can neutralize effectiveness of FIX to restore the patientsí clotting ability. We have also evaluated the presence of anti-FIX antibodies in hemophilia A patients using immunoassays that can detect neutralizing and non-neutralizing anti-FIX antibodies and that can be used to characterize these antibodies. Information on specificity of FIX inhibitors may be used to gain knowledge about the origin and consequences of an antibody response to FIX. The FIX molecule is a 55 kD glycoprotein with five domains, designated GLA, EGF-1, EGF-2, AP and SP, which have distinct roles in mediating FIX function. The AP (activation peptide) and the GLA (gamma-carboxylated) domains contain most post-translational modifications that are present on FIX. Samples from 12 inhibitor patients (treated with plasma-derived FIX) were evaluated for binding specificity to GLA and AP domains of FIX using peptides, variants, and mutants of recombinant FIX (rFIX). These antibodies bind similarly to rFIX and pdFIX. The 12 patients tested did not have any significant level of binding to the activation peptide region. In contrast, 7 of the 12 patients had a significant level of binding to a peptide containing the fully gamma-carboxylated sequence of the GLA domain. Some of the patients had anti-FIX antibodies that appeared to be directed only against the GLA region while the other 6 patients had intermediate levels of reactivity. The role that gamma-carboxylation plays in antibody binding to the GLA region was also examined. All patientsí antibodies bound similarly to rFIX and to a variant of FIX with 10 gamma-carboxyl groups. However, binding to an rFIX variant that had a very low number of gammacarboxyl groups was more variable. Some patientís anti-GLA antibodies required a high level of gammacarboxylation indicating that these antibodies are directed against the calcium-dependent conformation of FIX. These data suggest that anti-FIX antibodies that develop in hemophilia B patients are not directed against the AP domain while the GLA domain appears to be a major epitope for such antibodies. The fact that most patients antibodies were only partially reactive with the GLA domain suggests that additional epitopes exist on one or more other domains of the FIX molecule.

Contributors

Rachel T. Barrow, Department of Medicine, Emory University, Atlanta, GA

Ernest Briët, M.D., Departments of Internal Medicine and Pediatrics, Academic Medical Center, Amsterdam, The Netherlands

Linda C. Burkly, Ph.D., Biogen, Inc., Cambridge, MA

Bianca M. Conti-Fine, M.D., Department of Biochemistry, Molecular Biology, and Biophysics, Department of Pharmacology, University of Minnesota, Minneapolis-St. Paul,

Brenda M. Diethelm-Okita, Department of Biochemistry, Molecular Biology, and Biophysics, University of Minnesota, Minneapolis-St. Paul, MN

Jeffrey Frelinger, Ph.D., Department of Microbiology and Immunology, University of North Carolina at Chapel Hill, Chapel Hill, NC

James N. George, Department of Medicine, Hematology-Oncology Section, University of Oklahoma Health Sciences Center, Oklahoma City, OK

Roberta Greenwood, Department of Microbiology and Immunology, University of North Carolina at Chapel Hill, Chapel Hill, NC

A. Gringeri, Angelo Bianchi Bonomi Hemophilia and Thrombosis Center and the IRCCS Maggiore Hospital and University of Milan, Milan, Italy

John F. Healey, Department of Medicine, Emory University, Atlanta, GA

Ulla Hedner, M.D. Novo Nordisk A/S, Malov, Denmark and University of Lund, Lund Sweden

Katherine High, M.D., Department of Pediatrics, University of Pennsylvania School of Medicine, The Children's Hospital of Philadelphia, Philadelphia, PA

Marc G. Jacquemin, Center for Molecular and Vascular Biology, University of Leuven, Leuven, Belgium

Rima F. Jubran, M.D., Department of Hematology/Oncology, Childrens Hospital, National Medical Center, Washington, D.C.

Michael Kalafatis, Ph.D., Department of Chemistry, Cleveland State University, Cleveland, and Department of Molecular Cardiology, Lerner Research Institute, Cleveland Clinic Foundation, Cleveland OH

Nigel S. Key, Department of Medicine, University of Minnesota, Minneapolis-St. Paul, MN

Mark Krampf, Department of Biochemistry, Molecular Biology, and Biophysics, University of Minnesota, Minneapolis-St. Paul, MN

Peter J. Larson, M.D., Department of Pediatrics, University of Pennsylvania School of Medicine, The Children's Hospital of Philadelphia, Philadelphia, PA

Pete Lollar, M.D., Department of Medicine, Emory University, Atlanta, GA

Naomi L.C. Luban, M.D., Department of Transfusion Medicine, Childrens Hospital, National Medical Center, Washington, D.C.

Kenneth G. Mann, Ph.D., Department of Biochemistry, College of Medicine, University of Vermont, Burlington, VT

Pier M. Mannucci, M.D., Angelo Bianchi Bonomi Hemophilia and Thrombosis Center and the IRCCS Maggiore Hospital and University of Milan, Milan, Italy

L. Mendolicchio, Angelo Bianchi Bonomi Hemophilia and Thrombosis Center and the IRCCS Maggiore Hospital and University of Milan, Milan, Italy

Alan T. Nurden, Ph.D., Laboratoire de Pathologie Cellulaire de l' Hémostase, Hôpital Cardiologique, Pessac, France

Paquita Nurden, Laboratoire de Pathologie Cellulaire de l' Hémostase, Hôpital Cardiologique, Pessac, France

David K. Okita, Department of Biochemistry, Molecular Biology, and Biophysics, University of Minnesota, Minneapolis-St. Paul, MN

Ernest T. Parker, Department of Medicine, Emory University, Atlanta, GA

Marjolein Peters, Departments of Internal Medicine and Pediatrics, Academic Medical Center, Amsterdam, The Netherlands

Mark T. Redding, Department of Biochemistry, Molecular Biology, and Biophysics, Department of Medicine, University of Minnesota, Minneapolis-St. Paul, MN

Jean-Marie R. Saint-Remy, M.D., Ph.D., Center for Molecular and Vascular Biology, University of Leuven, Leuven, Belgium

Beatrijs Vanzieleghem, Center for Molecular and Vascular Biology, University of Leuven, Leuven, Belgium

Huiyun Wu, Department of Biochemistry, Molecular Biology, and Biophysics, University of Minnesota, Minneapolis-St. Paul, MN

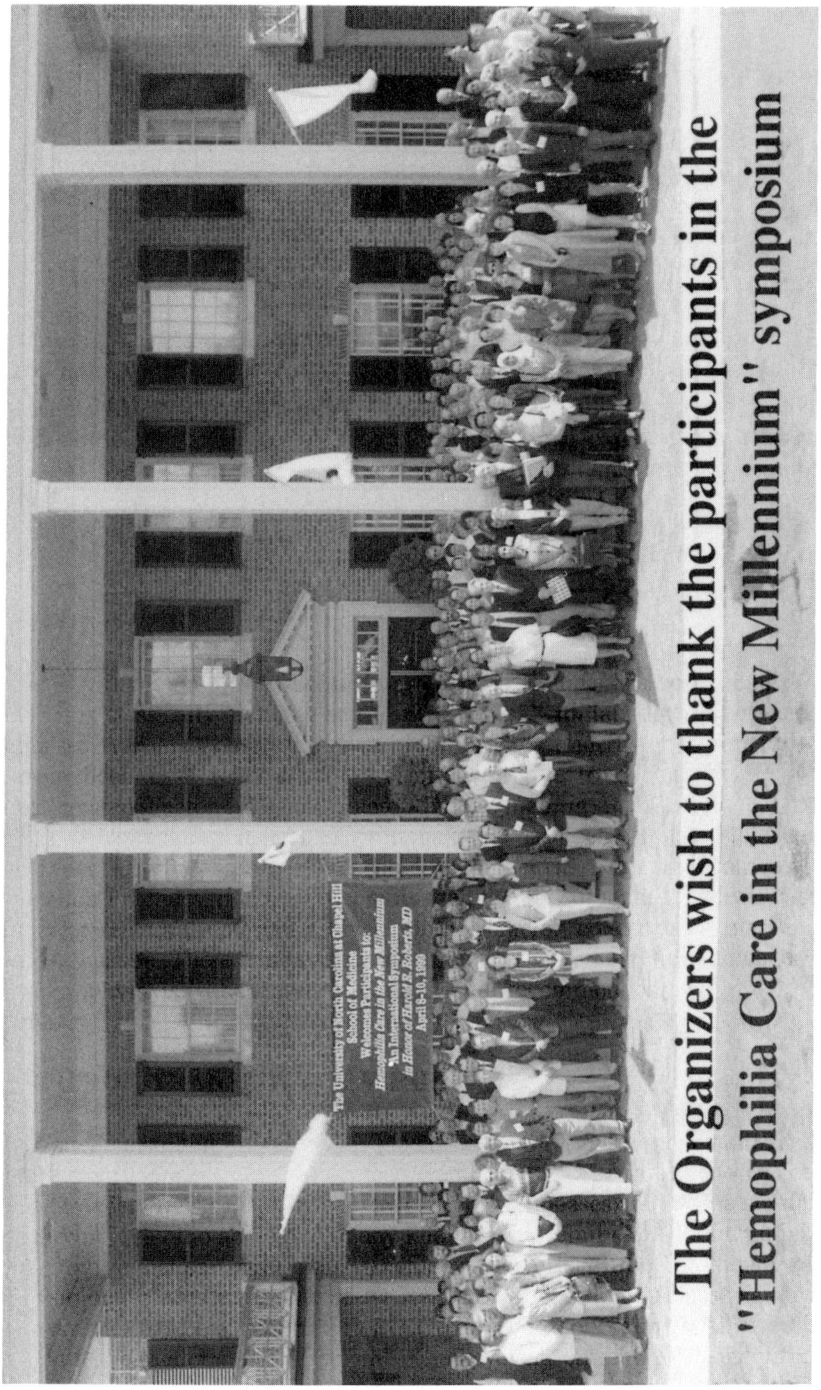
The University of North Carolina at Chapel Hill
School of Medicine
Welcomes Participants to:
Hemophilia Care in the New Millennium
An International Symposium
in Honor of Harold R. Roberts, MD
April 8-10, 1999
The Organizers wish to thank the participants in the
"Hemophilia Care in the New Millennium" symposium

INDEX